KT-386-939

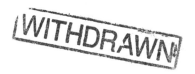
WITHDRAWN

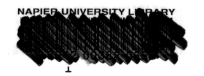
NAPIER UNIVERSITY LIBRARY

A Colour Atlas of the
Digestive System

A Colour Atlas of the
DIGESTIVE SYSTEM

Roy E. Pounder
MA, MD, FRCP
Reader in Medicine
Academic Department of Medicine
Royal Free Hospital School of Medicine
London

Miles C. Allison
MB, MRCP
Research Fellow and Honorary Lecturer in Medicine
Academic Department of Medicine
Royal Free Hospital School of Medicine
London

Amar P. Dhillon
MA, MD, MRCP, MRCPath
Senior Lecturer in Histopathology
Department of Histopathology
Royal Free Hospital School of Medicine
London

LIBRARY
NORTH LOTHIAN COLLEGE
OF NURSING & MIDWIFERY
13 CREWE ROAD SOUTH
EDINBURGH EH4 2LD

Wolfe Medical Publications Ltd

616.3075 Pou

Copyright © R.E. Pounder, M.C. Allison, A.P. Dhillon, 1989
First published 1989 by Wolfe Medical Publications Ltd
Printed by W.S. Cowell Ltd, Ipswich, England
ISBN 0 7234 0886 6

All rights reserved. No reproduction, copy or transmission of this
publication may be made without written permission.

No part of this publication may be reproduced, copied or
transmitted save with written permission or in accordance with the
provisions of the Copyright Act 1956 (as amended), or under the terms of
any licence permitting limited copying issued by the Copyright Licensing
Agency, 33-34 Alfred Place, London, WC1E 7DP.

Any person who does any unauthorised act in relation to this publication
may be liable to criminal prosecution and civil claims for damages.

A CIP catalogue record for this book is available from the British Library.

This book is one of the titles in the series of Wolfe Medical Atlases, a series
that brings together the world's largest systematic published collection of
diagnostic colour photographs.

For a full list of Atlases in the series, plus forthcoming titles and details of
our surgical, dental and veterinary Atlases, please write to Wolfe Medical
Publications Ltd, 2-16 Torrington Place, London WC1E 7LT, England.

Contents

DEDICATION

To Christine, Caroline and Gouri

Acknowledgements

We gratefully acknowledge the generosity of the following colleagues, who provided illustrations for this atlas.

CHAPTER 1
Mrs Gwen Chessell (**3**), Dr D. MacDonald Burns (**6**), Dr H. Dodd (**10**), Dr S. R. Smith (**15**).

CHAPTER 3
Dr G. E. Griffin (**47**), Dr F. Warwick (**49**), Dr B. Dean (**58**, **59**), Dr M. J. Gallant (**61**), Dr A. Deery (**66**), Mr R. M. Kirk (**68**), Dr S. Lucas (**74**), Dr D. S. Ridley (**75**), Dr F. Warwick (**81**), Dr B. Dean (**83**), Professor K. E. F. Hobbs (**88**), Dr A. K. Burroughs (**92**, **93**).

CHAPTER 5
Dr A. B. Price (**126**), Professor Dame Sheila Sherlock (**156**), Dr A. Deery (**169**), Dr S. G. Bown (**151**, **152**, **200**), Mr R. M. Kirk (**198**, **199**), Dr R. Teague (**183**).

CHAPTER 6
Dr H. Adams (**215**), Mr R. M. Kirk (**262**. **263**).

CHAPTER 7
Dr L. K. Trejdoziewicz (**278**). Mr B. Chalk (**274**).

CHAPTER 8
Professor A. V. Hoffbrand (**281**), Dr L. K. Trejdoziewicz (**286**, **287**), Dr H. Dodd (**291**), Dr J. Crow (**300**, **301**, **302**, **303**), Dr F. Warwick (**306**), Dr L. Papadaki (**313**, **349**), Dr A. J. W. Hilson (**325**, **330**), Professor K. E. F. Hobbs (**329**), Mr R. M. Kirk (**339**).

CHAPTER 11
Dr L. K. Trejdoziewicz (**413**), Dr S. G. Bown (**420**, **421**), Dr M. J. Gallant (**437**, **438**), Dr E. Sweet (**446**), Surgeon Commander R. J. Leicester (**448**).

CHAPTER 12
Mr W. J. Dinning (**488**), Mrs Gwen Chessell (**489**), Dr S. H. Saverymuttu (**501**), Dr H. Adams (**510**).

CHAPTER 15
Dr F. Warwick (**576**), Dr P. Chiodini (**584**, **589**, **599**, **634**), Mr J. E. Williams (**591**, **592**, **595**, **596**), Dr J. Crow (**594**, **598**), Dr G. C. Cook (**603**), Dr R. T. D. Emond (**607**), Dr C. Farthing (**625**, **626**), Dr G. E. Griffin (**629**).

Introduction

A Colour Atlas of the Digestive System takes the reader from the top to the bottom of the alimentary tract—from diseases of the mouth and tongue to perianal disorders, via the oesophagus, stomach, and small and large bowel. It also describes the normal and diseased pancreas, but leaves the liver and biliary system to *A Colour Atlas of Liver Disease*, by Dame Sheila Sherlock and John Summerfield (Wolfe Medical Publications, 1979).

The main aim of *A Colour Atlas of the Digestive System* is to provide a wealth of clear illustrations of the gut in health and disease—each with a short and informative explanation to support diagnosis and thus complement a standard textbook of gastroenterology such as *Diseases of the Gut and Pancreas*, edited by J. J. Misiewicz, R. E. Pounder and C. W. Venables (Blackwell Scientific Publications, 1987). We have taken advantage of the modern investigative techniques—such as fibreoptic endo-scopy, computerised tomography, monoclonal antibodies, scanning electron microscopy—and describe the latest diseases: AIDS, *Campylobacter pylori* gastritis and cryptosporidiosis.

Many of the images in this book have been collected from the everyday clinical activity at the Royal Free Hospital over the past four years. However, we would not have been able to compile this book without extra help from colleagues. Our particular thanks go to Dr R. Dick, Dr S. Lucas, Dr J. Rode, Dr D. Brew, and Mr A. A. M. Lewis, all of whom loaned even more slides than those listed in the Acknowledgements. Our grateful thanks for photographic help go to Mr F. Moll (Department of Morbid Anatomy) and Mrs Ann K. Sym and her colleagues in the Department of Medical Illustration of the Royal Free Hospital School of Medicine. We are particularly indebted to Mrs Julia Young, who prepared the manuscript.

CHAPTER 1

Diseases of the Mouth and Tongue

1

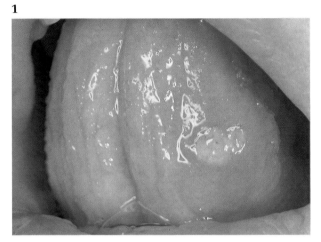

2

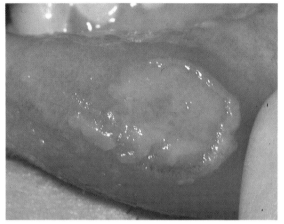

1 Aphthous ulcers. These can occur anywhere in the oral cavity, and are more common in women. Although they usually occur in isolation, their presence may be associated with poor dental hygiene, iron deficiency, folate and vitamin B_{12} deficiency, coeliac disease, Crohn's disease or ulcerative colitis. They also occur in healthy individuals for no apparent reason.

2 Large aphthous ulcer of the lower lip. Major aphthous ulcers of this kind are usually solitary rather than multiple, and they heal more slowly than minor aphthous ulcers. Both types tend to recur. The management includes treatment of nutritional deficiencies, topical analgesia and topical corticosteroids.

3

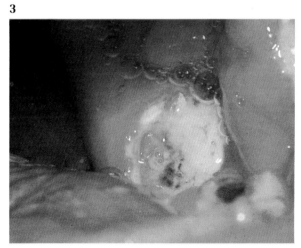

4

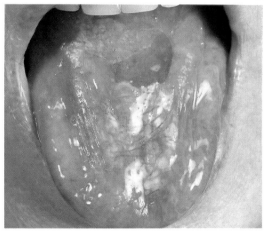

3 Behçet's syndrome. This is a rare chronic relapsing disorder with uveitis, and ulceration of the mouth and genitalia. The pathology of the ulcers is similar to that of aphthous ulceration. Occasionally the central nervous system and lower gastrointestinal tract may be involved. The oral lesions are treated in the same manner as recurrent aphthous ulcers.

4 Lichen planus of the tongue is often associated with violaceous papules that characteristically occur on the front of the wrists, in the lumbar region or around the ankles. Although the skin lesions usually heal after several months, mucous membrane involvement may persist for years, although it is often asymptomatic and may be noticed first by a dentist during routine examination.

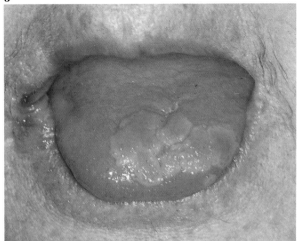

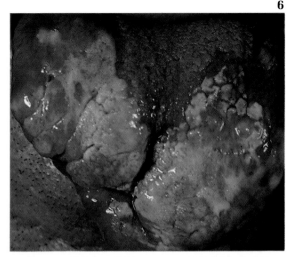

5 Condylomata acuminata of the tongue. This papillomatous growth can occur in the mouth, anogenital skin or mucous membranes. It is often the result of anogenital transmission of a papovavirus. The involved tongue may have a cauliflower-like surface, as in this example. Sessile or pedunculated condylomatous polyps may develop. Surgical excision is only rarely followed by recurrence. In addition, the patient in this photograph has angular cheilitis (see also **10** and **53**).

6 Leucoplakia of the tongue. Whitish patches of the tongue or buccal mucosa that cannot be removed by scraping are termed leucoplakia. Although there is usually no known cause, syphilis or candidal infections can give rise to this appearance. These lesions should be biopsied, as they may contain epithelial atypia or squamous carcinoma.

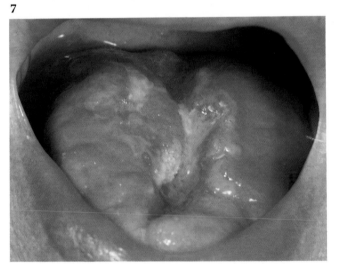

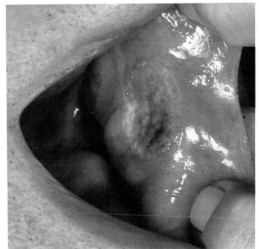

7 Carcinoma of the tongue may follow leucoplakia or submucous fibrosis (a condition seen in the Far East, related to eating chillies). Lesions of this kind may require wide local excision. Radiotherapy may be useful in inoperable cases.

8 Carcinoma of the mouth is histologically a squamous carcinoma. Causative factors are the same as for carcinoma of the tongue, and include pipe smoking, tobacco chewing, alcohol consumption, and chronic dental and oral infection, as well as leucoplakia and submucous fibrosis. After establishing the diagnosis by biopsy, surgical excision with block dissection of the regional lymph nodes (with or without radiotherapy) is required. Radiotherapy is useful for inoperable tumours and as a primary treatment for lip cancer.

9   Geographic tongue, or erythema migrans, is usually manifested by a patch of erythema with well-defined edges affecting the dorsum of the tongue. It is often asymptomatic and requires no treatment.

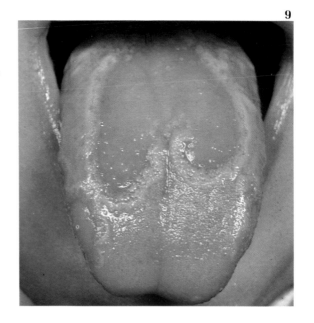

9

10   Hereditary haemorrhagic telangiectasia (Osler–Rendu–Weber syndrome). This condition is dominantly inherited, and usually presents in puberty or later. Multiple telangiectases occur in the skin and mucous membranes. Patients usually present with nose bleeds or iron deficiency anaemia as a result of bleeding from lesions in the gastrointestinal tract. This patient also has angular stomatitis on the right side.

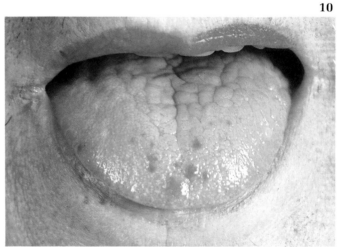

10

11   Hereditary haemorrhagic telangiectasia of the stomach, seen on endoscopic inspection of the gastric fundus. The telangiectasia in the gastrointestinal tract may be asymptomatic. They may present with either acute gastrointestinal haemorrhage or iron deficiency anaemia as a result of recurrent bleeding. Surgery, laser therapy or electrocautery may be necessary to control the haemorrhage, but further lesions may develop elsewhere.

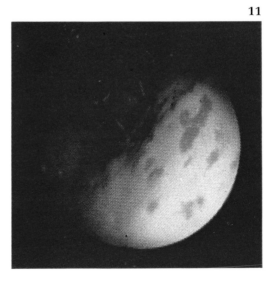

11

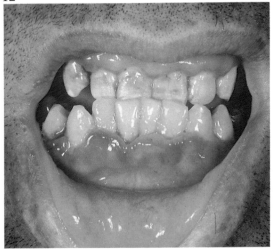

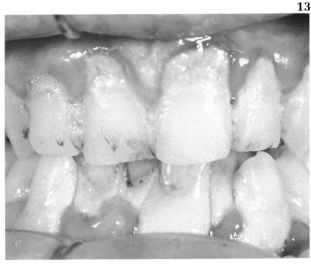

12   Scurvy is due to lack of vitamin C (ascorbic acid). The gums have a swollen, spongy appearance which may lead to necrosis and bleeding. The skin may show keratosis and plugging of hair follicles with capillary congestion and haemorrhage. The condition can also present with poor wound healing.

13   Gingivitis is usually caused by dental plaque which accumulates as a result of poor dental hygiene. The plaque is colonised by Gram-positive and Gram-negative organisms, and by anaerobic bacteria. Chronic gingival inflammation may result in breakdown of the periodontal membrane with loss of supporting bone, which may necessitate complete dental extraction.

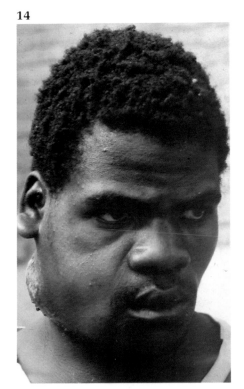

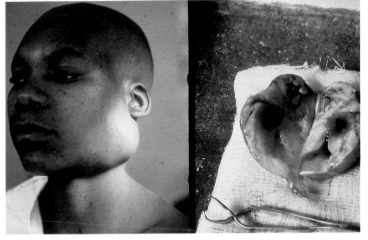

14   Parotid abscess usually results from ascending infection of the parotid gland. Treatment is by drainage of the abscess through an incision at the point of maximal tenderness under general anaesthesia. It is a rare complication of poor oral hygiene in very ill patients.

15   Salivary tumours. The most common salivary tumour is the pleomorphic salivary adenoma. These lesions require superficial parotidectomy and, although they are benign, they frequently recur as multiple nodules. Frank carcinoma of the salivary glands is uncommon, but this tumour may invade neighbouring structures such as skin, bone or facial nerve.

CHAPTER 2

The Normal Oesophagus

This hollow structure, about 25 cm long, is responsible for the propulsion of food boluses and liquid from the pharynx and down to the stomach. It is lined by non-keratinised, stratified squamous epithelium, to protect it from heat, cold and mechanical insult. The epithelial layer and submucosa are surrounded by longitudinal and circular smooth muscle fibres, and these are responsible for peristalsis. The oesophagus is a posterior mediastinal structure, lying anterior to the vertebral column but posterior to the trachea and the origins of the right and left main bronchi. The middle third of the oesophagus is closely related to the arch of the aorta, and the lower oesophagus lies behind the heart.

The arterial supply to the cervical oesophagus derives from the inferior thyroid arteries. The thoracic oesophagus is supplied by branches from the descending aorta, bronchial arteries and right posterior intercostal arteries. The lowest portion of the oesophagus is supplied by the left gastric and inferior phrenic arteries. Venous drainage is into the inferior thyroid, azygos and left gastric veins. The lower oesophagus forms an anastomosis between the portal venous system (via the left gastric vein) and the systemic venous system (via the azygos vein); this anastomotic link is of major clinical importance in the sequelae of portal hypertension. There is a rich lymphatic drainage. Nerve supply is from branches of the recurrent laryngeal nerves and sympathetic trunks in the neck. The thoracic oesophagus is supplied by branches of the vagus nerve, and parasympathetic and sympathetic fibres form a plexus around the oesophagus.

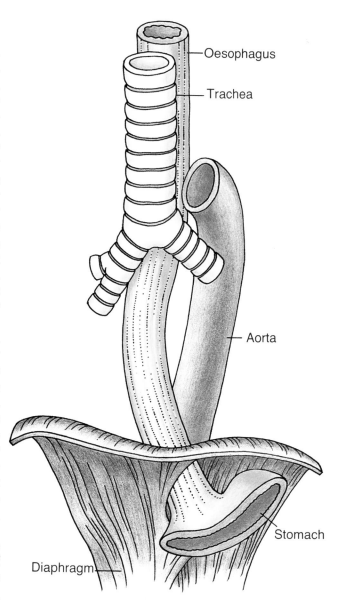

The lower oesophageal sphincter is a physiological barrier to reflux of gastric contents into the oesophagus. It is controlled by fibres arising from the vagus nerve and coeliac plexus.

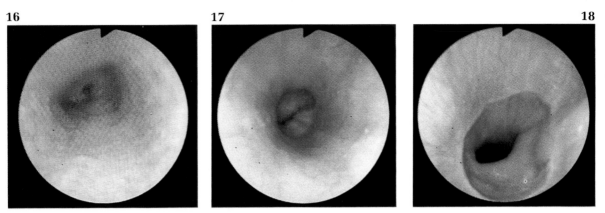

16   Endoscopic view of the middle oesophagus. The shiny pink squamous epithelium of the oesophagus is seen.

17   Peristalsis in the normal oesophagus, shown on endoscopy. Peristalsis is provoked by oesophageal distension or swallowing. The peristaltic waves pass from the pharynx to the lower oesophageal sphincter at a speed of about 3 cm/s.

18   Gastro-oesophageal junction. An endoscopic view of the junction between the pink (squamous) oesophageal epithelium and the red (columnar) gastric mucous membrane.

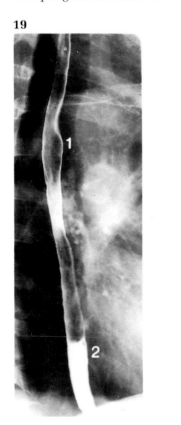
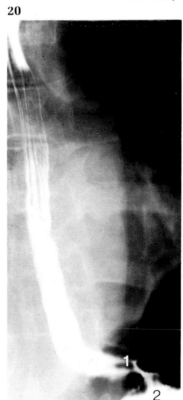
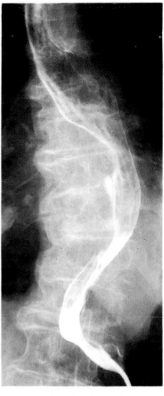

19   Normal barium swallow. This lateral view shows an empty undistended oesophagus. The upper oesophagus lies behind the trachea and left main bronchus (1). The lower oesophagus is separated from the left atrium by the pericardium (2).

20   Normal barium swallow. This oblique view shows the lower oesophagus draining barium via the gastro-oesophageal junction (1) into the stomach just below the left diaphragm (2).

21   Displacement of the normal oesophagus by an enlarged left atrium in a patient with severe mitral stenosis. This displacement is usually asymptomatic, but ulceration may develop in patients taking slow-release potassium supplements.

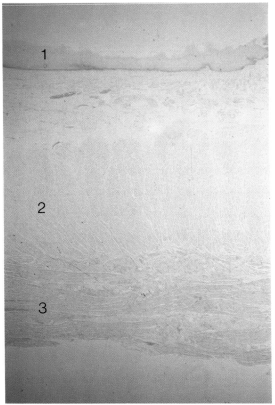

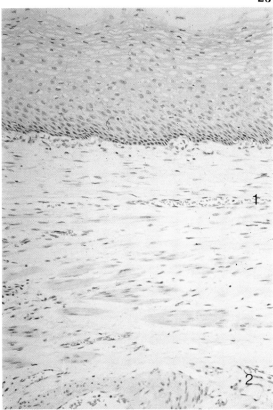

22 **Normal oesophagus** in longitudinal section: squamous epithelium (1) overlies the connective tissue of the submucosa and the thick circular (2) and longitudinal (3) muscle coats.

23 **Normal oesophagus** is lined by squamous epithelium and underlying connective tissue. The epithelium shows its normal orderly maturation, and the strands of smooth muscle in the connective tissue separate the lamina propria above (1) from the submucosa below (2).

24 **Gastro-oesophageal junction.** This photomicrograph shows the sudden change from the squamous epithelium of the oesophagus (1) and the glandular columnar epithelium of the gastric cardia (2). The junction shows a little chronic inflammation, but is otherwise normal.

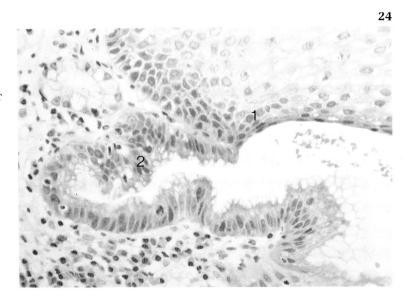

CHAPTER 3

Diseases of the Oesophagus

25

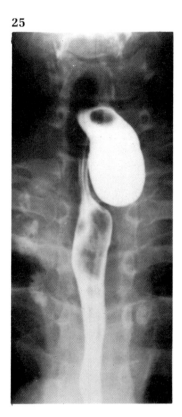

26

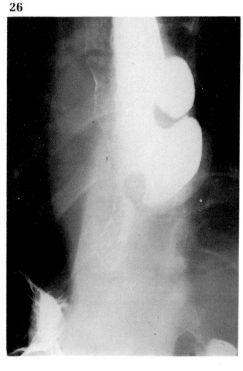

27

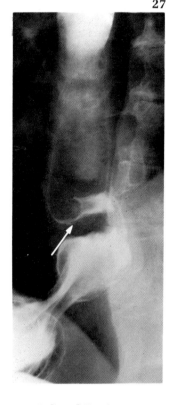

25   Pharyngeal pouch, demonstrated on barium swallow x-ray. A pouch arises between the cricopharyngeal sphincter and the inferior constrictor muscle, and it may present with intermittent dysphagia, food regurgitation or pulmonary aspiration. Endoscopic examination may be hazardous in such patients, as perforation of the diverticulum may occur.

26   Oesophageal diverticula. These mid- or lower oesophageal diverticula are caused by abnormal motility. Mid-oesophageal diverticula may be due to traction by adjacent mediastinal inflammation—for example, tuberculosis involving the peribronchial lymph nodes.

27   Schatzki's rings occur in the lower oesophagus (arrow) and are usually asymptomatic. Occasionally they present with intermittent dysphagia or bolus obstruction, and in these circumstances may require dilatation.

28 | **29**

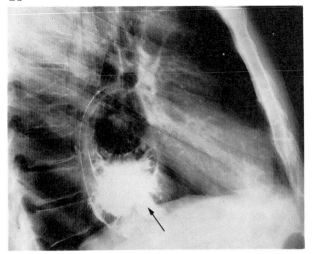 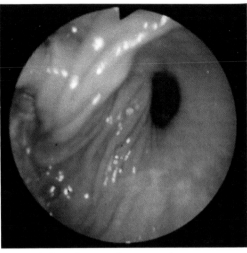

28 Sliding hiatus hernia (arrow), demonstrated on this lateral view during a barium swallow. The upper stomach lies within the thoracic cavity above the diaphragm. Hiatus hernias are usually asymptomatic, but they may be associated with symptoms of oesophageal reflux, oesophagitis or stricture formation. The treatment includes avoidance of smoking, advice on timing and size of meals, and weight reduction. Drugs which inhibit gastric acid secretion are valuable in the treatment of reflux oesophagitis in these patients. Surgical treatment is required rarely.

29 Sliding hiatus hernia. This endoscopic photograph was taken within the hiatus hernia sac. The oesophago-gastric junction lies within the thoracic cavity, above the level of the diaphragmatic hiatus.

30 Rolling hiatus hernia. In this variety of hiatus hernia the fundus of the stomach is found within the thoracic cavity, adjacent to the lower oesophagus. The barium meal shows the para-oesophageal hernia (large arrow) and the level of the diaphragmatic hiatus (small arrow).

30 | **31**

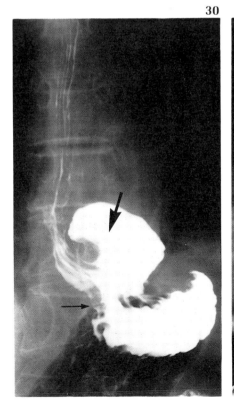 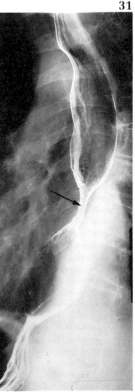

31 Benign oesophageal stricture. This double-contrast barium swallow demonstrates a smooth lower oesophageal stricture (arrow) above a hiatus hernia. These strictures probably result from oesophagitis caused by acid reflux into the lower oesophagus. They are usually seen in older patients presenting with gradually developing dysphagia associated with heartburn.

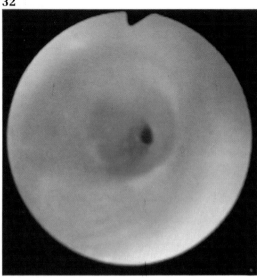

32 Endoscopic view of a benign oesophageal stricture. This very tight stricture was the result of long-standing oesophagitis. The surrounding mucosa is smooth, but reddened due to oesophagitis. Benign strictures may be dilated endoscopically using oesophageal dilators (**33** and **34**).

33

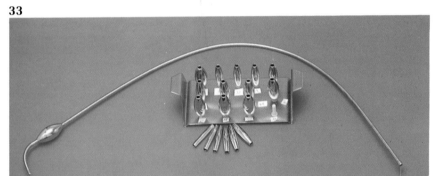

33 Eder–Peustow dilators. The dilatation of benign oesophageal strictures is carried out by passing a guide wire through the stricture into the stomach under direct endoscopic vision and using x-ray screening. The endoscope is then removed and the metal olives are passed over the guide wire and through the stricture. Olives of increasing size are used until dilatation has been achieved.

34

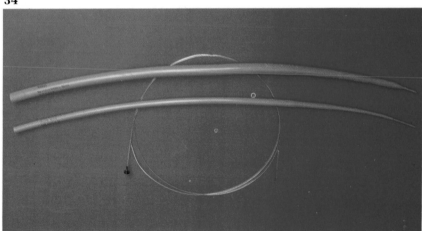

34 Celestin oesophageal dilators. These graduated dilators may be used as an alternative to Eder–Peustow dilators (**33**) for the management of benign oesophageal strictures. The strictures tend to recur with either technique, and symptomatic patients may require frequent dilatations.

35 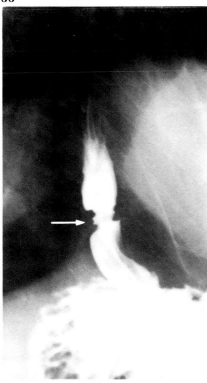 **36** 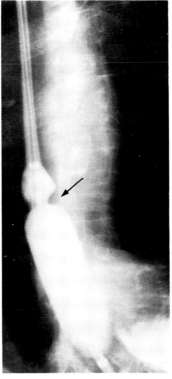 **37**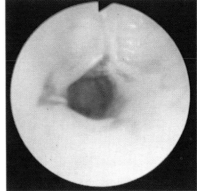

37   Mild linear oesophagitis and oesophageal stricture. This endoscopic view demonstrates slight asymptomatic narrowing of the lower oesophagus with streaky linear oesophagitis above the stricture.

35 and **36   Benign oesophageal stricture (35)** dilated under x-ray control (**36**) using a cylindrical balloon. This balloon is passed via the nose or mouth to the level of the stricture, and is inflated until the narrowing (arrowed) is seen to disappear.

38   Moderate ulcerating oesophagitis. This endoscopic view shows linear lower oesophageal ulcers and oesophagitis. The factors responsible for oesophagitis are not completely understood. Acid reflux into the oesophagus via a weak lower oesophageal sphincter is frequently responsible. Associations of oesophagitis include hiatus hernia, smoking and obesity. Although acid and pepsin from the stomach are usually implicated, bile reflux in patients after gastrectomy may lead to similar endoscopic appearances.

38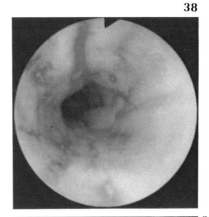

39   Severe ulcerating oesophagitis. This endoscopic view shows oesophagitis and confluent lower oesophageal ulceration. The treatment of oesophagitis is similar to that of the hiatus hernia, but drugs that control gastric acid secretion are important in controlling oesophagitis. Endoscopic biopsy and brush cytology should be performed to exclude malignancy in patients with severe oesophagitis.

39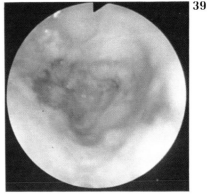

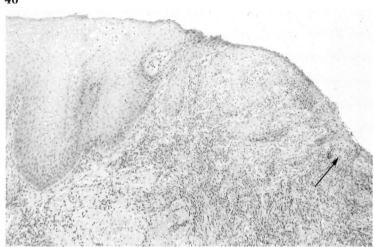

40 Gastro-oesophageal reflux has led to an inflamed and ulcerated oesophageal mucosa. The epithelium is thickened on the left, with an expansion of the basal layers. However, epithelial maturation remains orderly. The epithelium has been lost on the right, and a little attempted healing is seen at the ulcer edge (arrow). The base of the ulcer and the surrounding connective tissue show chronic inflammation.

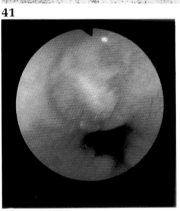

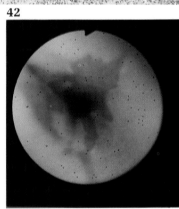

41 Oesophageal ulcer. This isolated lower oesophageal ulcer was seen in a patient taking a non-steroidal anti-inflammatory drug. Non-steroidal anti-inflammatory drugs are also associated with benign oesophageal stricture. Other drugs that have been implicated in oesophageal ulceration include emepronium bromide and slow-release potassium supplements. All tablets should be taken with plenty of water, with the patient sitting or standing.

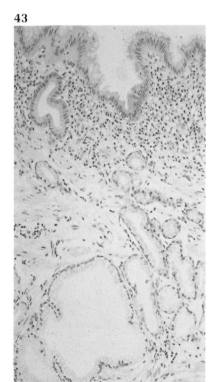

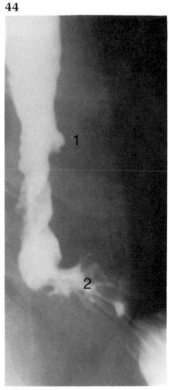

42 Barrett's oesophagus results from the replacement of the lower oesophageal epithelium with gastric columnar epithelium. This endoscopic view shows the irregular border between the two types of epithelium (compare with normal appearance in **18**). It is believed that this mucosal change may result from prolonged gastro-oesophageal reflux.

43 Barrett's oesophageal mucosa is histologically indistinguishable from gastric mucosa with non-specialised glands. The gland at the bottom of the figure shows cystic dilatation, and there is a little superficial chronic inflammation.

44 Barrett's ulcer, occurring within the lower oesophagus above the squamo-columnar junction. This barium swallow shows the ulcer crater (1) 5 cm above the oesophago-gastric junction (2).

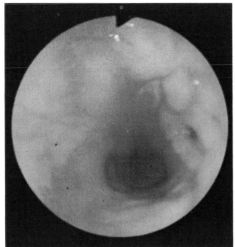

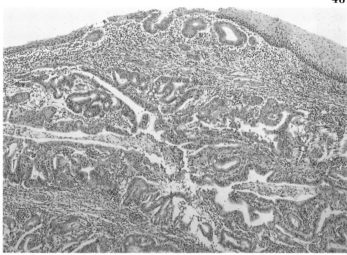

45   Barrett's ulcer, shown endoscopically (at 1 o'clock) above the squamo-columnar epithelial junction. Such ulcers should always be brushed and biopsied to exclude malignancy, as Barrett's oesophagus may undergo malignant transformation in approximately 10% of patients. The role of regular endoscopic screening for malignancy in patients with Barrett's oesophagus remains controversial.

46   Barrett's oesophagus: malignant transformation. Oesophageal squamous epithelium on the right changes abruptly to glandular epithelium. Infiltrative adenocarcinoma is seen underneath the dysplastic glandular epithelium.

47   Oral candidiasis. A severe example is seen here in a patient with the acquired immune deficiency syndrome (AIDS). The white patches of candidiasis may be seen anywhere within the oral cavity, but are found most commonly on the fauces. Predisposing factors include poor oral hygiene, immunosuppression, broad-spectrum antibiotic treatment and diabetes mellitus, as well as AIDS. The white plaques can be rubbed off with a swab, but the clinical appearance is so typical that microbiological confirmation is generally unnecessary.

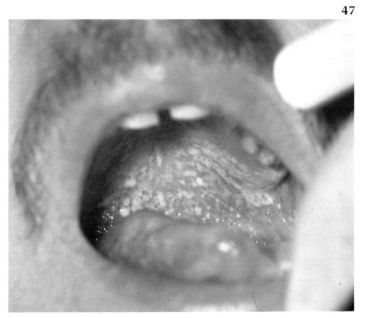

48

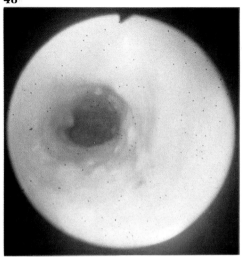

48 Oesophageal candidiasis, seen by endoscopy. This infection is usually asymptomatic and is often associated with oral candidiasis. Oesophageal candidiasis is common in patients who are immunosuppressed, in whom dysphagia and retrosternal discomfort may develop. In advanced cases the plaques of candidiasis may be confluent with frank mucosal ulceration. The fungal hyphae can be demonstrated microscopically in biopsies or brush cytology smears. The differential diagnosis includes reflux oesophagitis, *Cytomegalovirus* and *Herpes* virus infection.

49

50

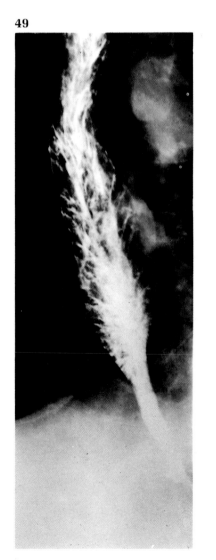

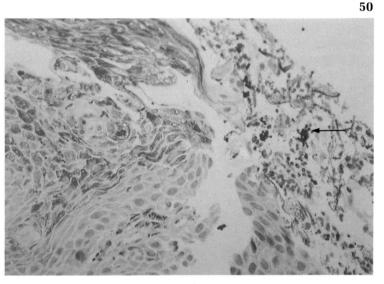

50 Oesophageal candidiasis. An oesophageal biopsy (stained with PAS) consisting of inflamed squamous epithelium and debris with dark red-staining colonies of *Candida* to the middle right of the field (arrow).

49 Oesophageal candidiasis, seen on barium swallow in a patient with dysphagia. The oesophageal mucosal irregularities seen on double-contrast barium radiology may be striking. In patients with human immunodeficiency virus infection (HIV) the presence of oesophageal candidiasis means that the patient has the full acquired immune deficiency syndrome (AIDS).

51

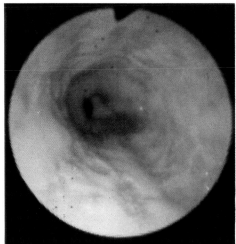

52

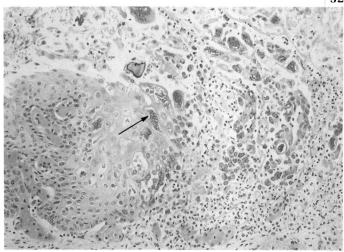

51 Herpes simplex oesophagitis may also occur in patients who are immunosuppressed or severely debilitated. Symptoms include severe dysphagia and haematemesis. Endoscopy demonstrates discrete or confluent superficial ulceration. A rise in complement-fixing antibodies against herpes simplex in the serum will confirm the diagnosis. Any biopsy must be performed cautiously, as there is a risk of viral transfer to the eyes of the endoscopist or assistant.

52 *Herpes simplex* oesophagitis. There is ulceration on the right. Epithelial cells within the inflammatory material and in the edge of the ulcer are multinucleate, and contain prominent nuclear inclusions (arrow).

53

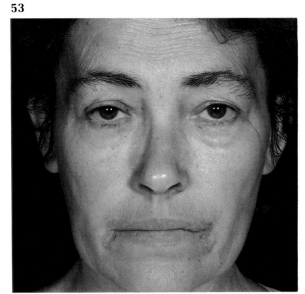

54

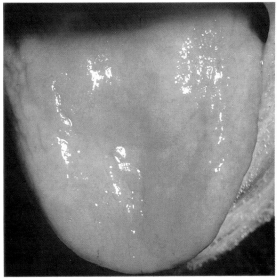

53 Iron deficiency anaemia. This patient has angular cheilitis and blue sclerae due to severe iron deficiency. This anaemia usually requires full gastroenterological investigation. The most common gastrointestinal causes include carcinoma or adenoma of the colon or stomach, oesophagitis, peptic ulceration, inflammatory bowel disease or coeliac disease.

54 Iron deficiency anaemia. Note the smooth tongue due to loss of papillae.

55

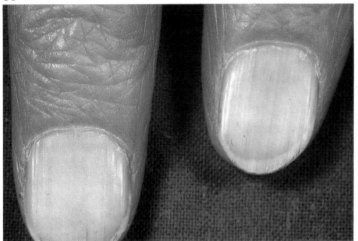

55 Iron deficiency anaemia. Early changes to the nails include brittleness and flattening. The pallor of the nail beds is a clue to the presence of anaemia.

56

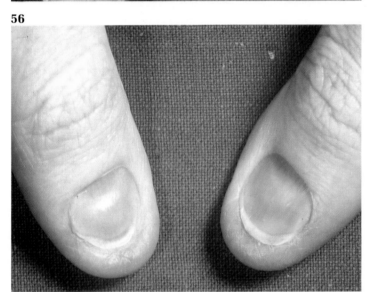

56 Koilonychia. Long-standing iron deficiency anaemia may produce brittle spoon-shaped nails.

57

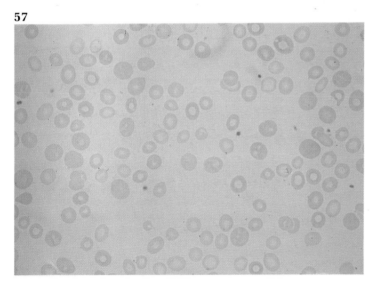

57 Iron deficiency anaemia. This blood film demonstrates variation in size and shape of the red cells (anisocytosis). Many of the red cells are small and pale (microcytic and hypochromic).

58   Oesophageal web. This barium swallow demonstrates the radiological appearance of a post-cricoid web (arrow). These develop from squamous epithelium and may progress to squamous carcinoma. The Patterson–Kelly or Plummer–Vinson syndrome includes intermittent dysphagia, glossitis, koilonychia and iron deficiency anaemia. This syndrome usually presents in post-menopausal women.

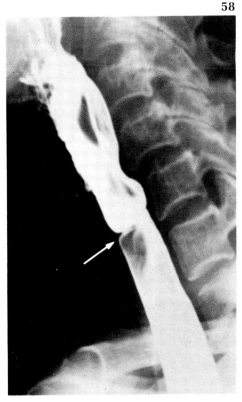
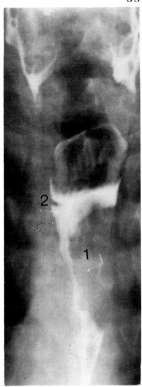

59   Oesophageal carcinoma (1) arising within an oesophageal web (2). This barium swallow was performed because of dysphagia, and it demonstrates a stricture caused by a large carcinoma arising at the site of an oesophageal web.

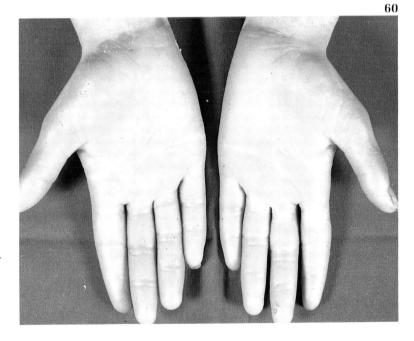

60   Tylosis palmaris. This hyperkeratosis of the palms of the hands (as well as the soles of the feet) has been associated with the presence of carcinoma of the oesophagus in two families.

NORTH LOTHIAN COLLEGE OF NURSING LIBRARY

61

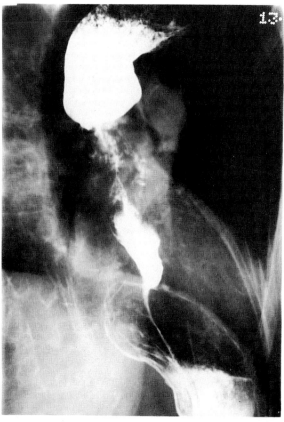

61 Oesophageal carcinoma typically presents with dysphagia, but may present with iron deficiency anaemia or dyspepsia. A barium swallow in this patient with dysphagia demonstrates a long, irregular stricture due to a carcinoma with dilatation of the oesophagus (filled with barium) above the stricture.

62

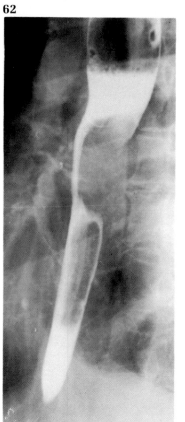

63

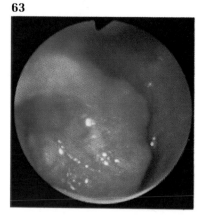

64

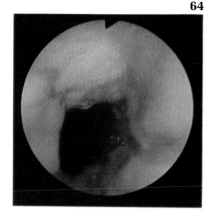

62 Oesophageal carcinoma. This barium swallow demonstrates a polypoid filling defect due to a carcinoma of the mid-oesophagus.

63 Oesophageal carcinoma, seen at endoscopy. The haemorrhagic polypoid carcinoma is seen within the oesophageal lumen. Oesophageal carcinomas are usually squamous, but an adenocarcinoma may occur in the lower oesophagus or spread upwards from the stomach.

64 Oesophageal carcinoma. An endoscopic view of a large malignant ulcer of the lower oesophagus. Biopsies taken from the edge of the ulcer confirmed squamous carcinoma.

65   Oesophageal carcinoma.
This post-mortem specimen
demonstrates a long polypoid
carcinoma and stricture.

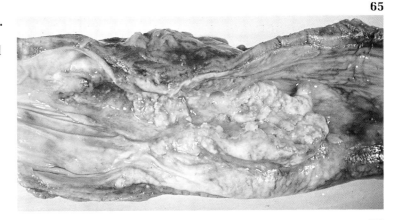

66   Oesophageal carcinoma. To
exclude malignancies,
endoscopic oesophageal brush
cytology and biopsy samples
should be taken from any area of
oesophageal ulceration. This
abnormal cytological smear was
obtained from a squamous
carcinoma of the oesophagus.

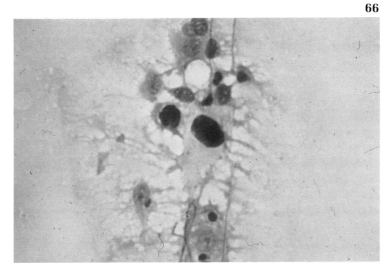

67   Oesophageal carcinoma. A
moderately differentiated
squamous cell carcinoma is seen,
infiltrating the base of an
oesophageal ulcer on the right and
the submucosa on the left.

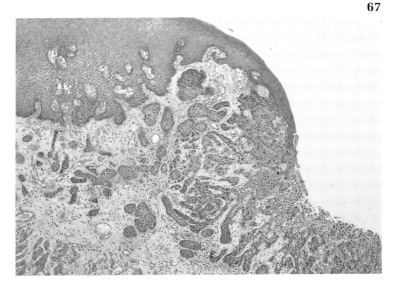

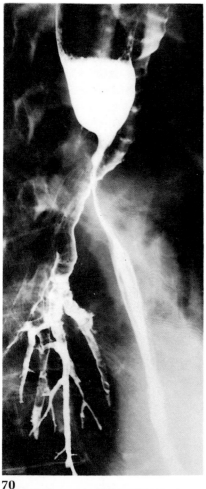

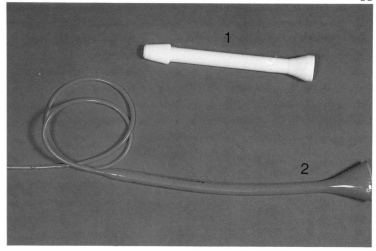

68 Tracheo-oesophageal fistula. This is an uncommon complication of oesophageal carcinoma (it more usually happens in the reverse direction, when a carcinoma of the bronchus extends into the oesophagus). A barium swallow demonstrates the malignant oesophageal stricture. Barium has entered the fistula and has opacified the bronchial tree. Oesophageal intubation is valuable in managing this complication (**69** and **70**).

69 Oesophageal carcinoma. The Atkinson tube (1) is inserted endoscopically, whereas the Mousseau–Barbin tube (2) is inserted surgically. They are useful in the palliation of dysphagia due to oesophageal carcinoma, as they allow swallowing of liquids and semi-solids. Similarly, endoscopic laser palliation may be useful in selected cases.

70

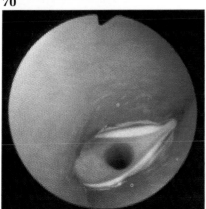

70 Atkinson tube, seen from above on endoscopy, after insertion for palliation of an oesophageal carcinoma.

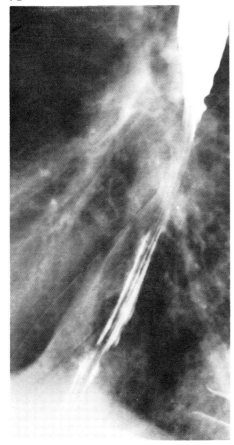

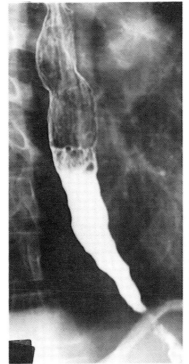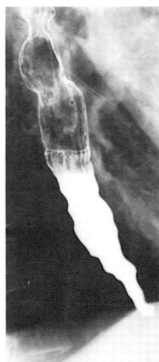

72   Achalasia. This disease of unknown origin results in failure of the lower oesophageal sphincter to relax. This barium swallow in a patient with achalasia demonstrates the typical smooth, tapered distal narrowing of the sphincter zone ('bird's beak'). Peristaltic contractions and retained barium are seen above the narrowing. Oesophagoscopy is advisable to exclude a carcinoma in such patients. Often the endoscope passes easily through the stricture into the stomach.

71   Extrinsic compression of the oesophagus. This barium swallow demonstrates a stricture of the mid-oesophagus, due to carcinoma of the bronchus. Other causes of extrinsic compression include mediastinal lymphadenopathy, retrosternal goitre and aortic aneurysm. This squamous carcinoma was treated with radiotherapy, which resulted in complete prolonged relief of dysphagia.

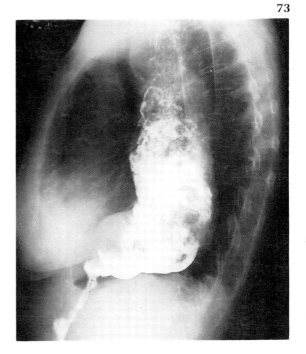

73   Achalasia. This gross example seen on barium swallow demonstrates marked dilatation of the oesophagus with food residue therein. Chronic pulmonary changes may result from recurrent aspiration. Approaches to treatment include pneumatic balloon dilatation and surgical cardiomyotomy (Heller's operation).

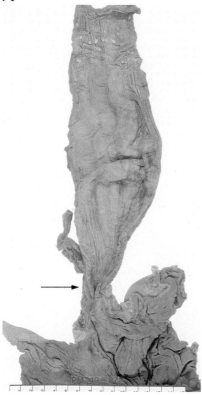

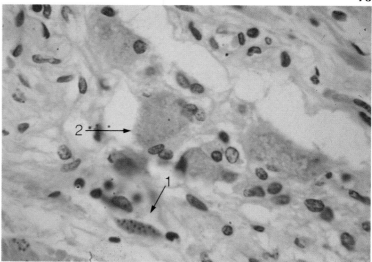

74   Achalasia. This post-mortem specimen demonstrates a dilated and flaccid oesophagus above the stricture (arrow).

75   Chagas' disease. This histological section demonstrates a pseudocyst of *Trypanosoma cruzi* (arrow 1) close to a degenerate nerve ganglion (arrow 2) in the oesophagus of a patient with Chagas' disease. The protozoan parasite may also affect the heart and hollow abdominal viscera. This disease is endemic in tropical South America, particularly Brazil. The disease may present with dysphagia or constipation (due to rectal involvement). The oesophageal form of the disease may present in a similar manner to achalasia.

76

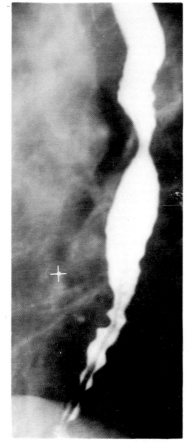

76   Corkscrew oesophagus. This barium swallow in a patient with dysphagia demonstrates a tortuous oesophagus due to disordered peristalsis. Manometry is valuable in defining the diffuse segmental oesophageal spasm in these patients. Oesophageal spasm may mimic angina pectoris, and the differential diagnosis is often difficult, as electrocardiographic abnormalities may be present in patients with oesophageal spasm. The treatment of this disorder is not clearly defined, although anticholinergic drugs and nifedipine may produce moderate improvement in some patients. Occasionally balloon dilatation or extended oesophageal surgical myotomy are required for severe symptoms due to oesophageal spasm.

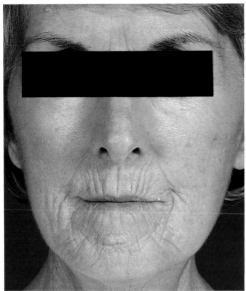

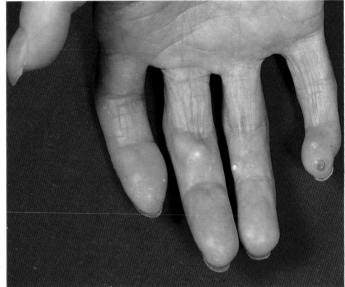

77   Systemic sclerosis. The facial appearance is typical. The skin around the mouth is tight, shiny and puckered. The patient's hands are shown in **78** and **79**.

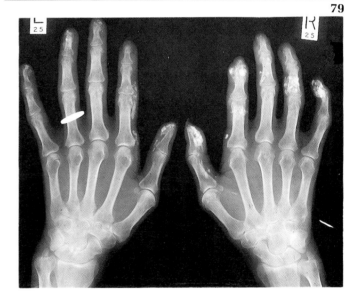

78 and 79   Systemic sclerosis. This patient (**77**) has the CREST variant of systemic sclerosis (*C*alcinosis, *R*aynaud's, o*E*sophageal disease, *S*clerodactyly, *T*elangiectasia). The hands of this patient (**78**) demonstrate the tethering of the skin (sclerodactyly) as well as nodules of the fingers due to calcinosis. This patient suffered from Raynaud's syndrome: prolonged episodes of digital vascular spasm have led to ulceration of the distal phalanx of the fifth digit. Telangiectasia of the skin is also present in this patient. Oesophageal involvement is the other part of this syndrome, which carries a better prognosis than systemic sclerosis. An x-ray of the hands of the patient (**79**) shows calcinosis and erosion of the terminal phalanges.

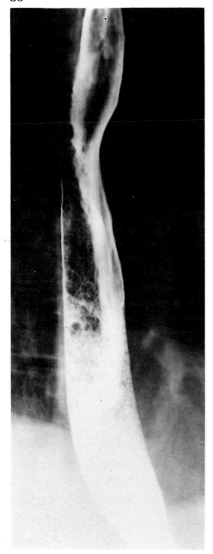

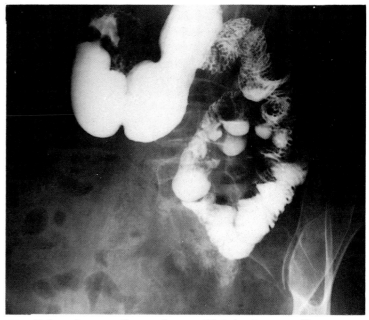

80   Scleroderma of oesophagus. This barium swallow demonstrates the smooth aperistaltic and dilated oesophagus resulting from the motility disorder of scleroderma. Patients with scleroderma, or the CREST syndrome, develop oesophageal smooth muscle atrophy and collagen replacement, leading to impaired oesophageal clearance. Severe reflux oesophagitis and stricture formation may result. These patients usually present with dysphagia which is notoriously difficult to treat. Treatment with an H_2-receptor antagonist may benefit patients with oesophageal reflux. Occasionally anti-reflux surgery is required.

81   Systemic sclerosis. This barium swallow demonstrates jejunal pseudo-diverticula containing air–contrast fluid levels. These result from small intestinal smooth muscle infiltration leading to markedly delayed small intestinal transit time and pseudo-obstruction. Malabsorption is common and may be exacerbated by small intestinal bacterial overgrowth, which can be controlled by orally-administered antibiotics. Pseudo-diverticula can also occur without systemic sclerosis.

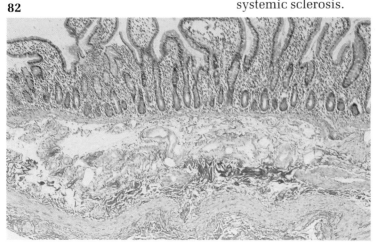

82   Systemic sclerosis. A biopsy of the small bowel from a patient with scleroderma. This section is stained with the van Gieson method, so that the excessive collagen representing the mural fibrosis characteristic of this condition is stained red.

83   Systemic sclerosis. This barium enema demonstrates the pseudo-diverticula (arrow) in a patient with widespread gastrointestinal infiltration. Small and large intestinal involvement with scleroderma is less common than oesophageal involvement. The haustral pattern disappears and the colon dilates with formation of saccules. The patient may become constipated and large-bowel obstruction may develop. The anal sphincter may also be involved.

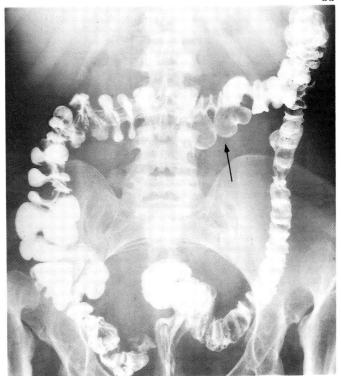

84   Oesophageal varices. This barium swallow demonstrates tortuous lower oesophageal and gastric varices in a patient with portal hypertension. Oesophageal varices usually present with haematemesis, which may be massive and life-threatening.

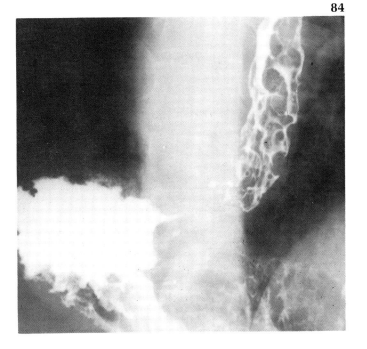

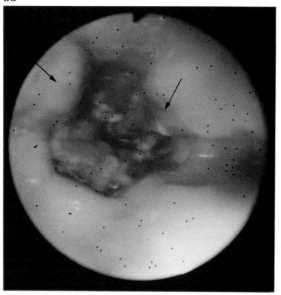

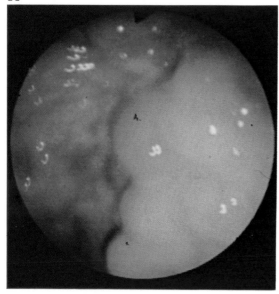

85 Oesophageal varices, seen on endoscopy. The blue submucous and subepithelial varices occur in the lower oesophagus and stomach (arrows). In patients with portal hypertension portal venous blood drains via the oesophageal veins and azygous vein into the superior vena cava.

86 Oesophageal varices. Huge lobulated venous saccules are seen here in the lower oesophagus by means of a side-viewing endoscope in a patient with cirrhosis due to primary sclerosing cholangitis.

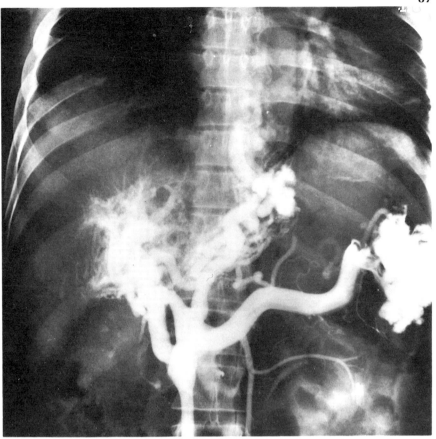

87 Oesophageal varices. This angiogram demonstrates the portal and splenic venous blood flowing into the oesophageal collaterals.

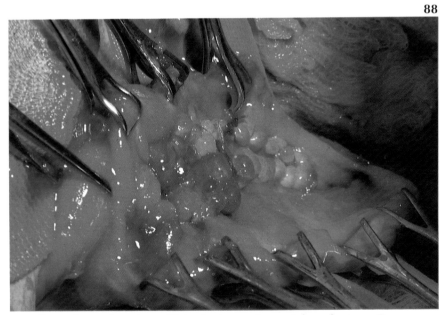

88 Oesophageal varices. This photograph was taken during a Boerema Crile transthoracic ligation of oesophageal varices. This particular operation is performed rarely nowadays.

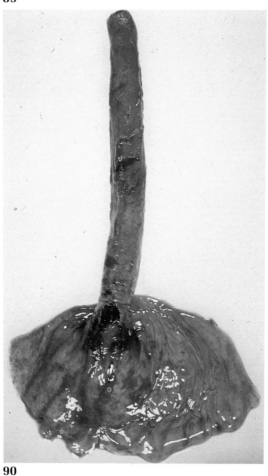

89 Oesophageal varices. This post-mortem oesophagus and stomach was obtained from a patient who had died from bleeding oesophageal varices. The specimen has been pulled inside out. Blood clot is visible in the upper stomach. The relationship of the varices to the oesophageal mucosa is seen.

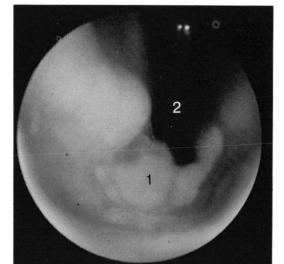

90 Gastric varices, seen in the cardia (1) on inversion of the endoscope (2).

91   Bleeding gastric varix. This transhepatic portogram shows the gastric varix oozing contrast into the stomach (arrow). Oesophageal tamponade with a Sengstaken–Blakemore tube had failed to control the haemorrhage. The gastric balloon of the Sengstaken–Blakemore tube is seen here as a circular lucency overlying the bleeding point. Transhepatic sclerosis of this collateral successfully controlled the haemorrhage for this patient, who was too ill for surgical intervention.

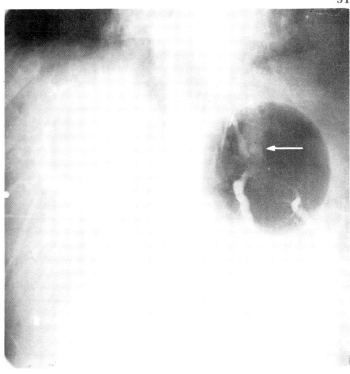

92   Bleeding oesophageal varix. Venous blood is seen here spurting from the bleeding varix at 3 o'clock on this endoscopic view.

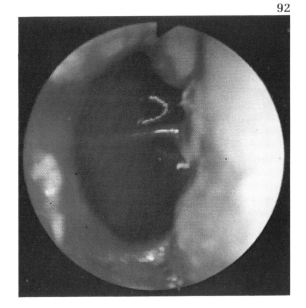

93

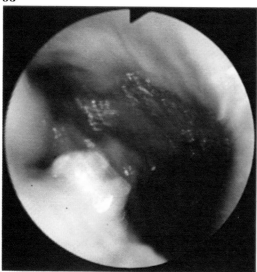

93 Gastric varices. Endoscopy shows a pale yellow fibrin plaque (the so-called 'white nipple sign') overlying a gastric varix that had bled recently. Stale blood clot is also seen in the stomach.

94

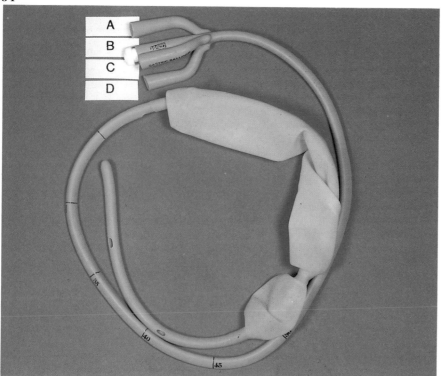

A
B
C
D

94 Sengstaken–Blakemore tube. This tube is used to control oesophageal variceal haemorrhage by means of balloon tamponade. Pressure by means of channel A inflates the oesophageal balloon. Air is introduced into channel B to inflate the gastric balloon in order to prevent displacement of the oesophageal balloon. Channels C (gastric aspiration) and D (oesophageal aspiration) enable blood and secretion to be sucked out.

95 Oesophageal varices. This view shows endoscopic injection sclerotherapy, which is valuable in controlling haemorrhage from oesophageal varices.

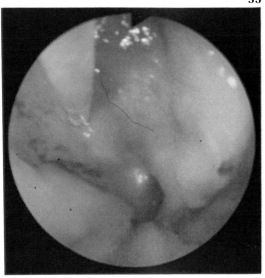

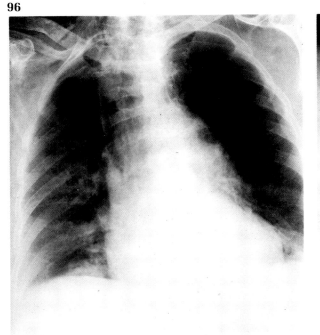

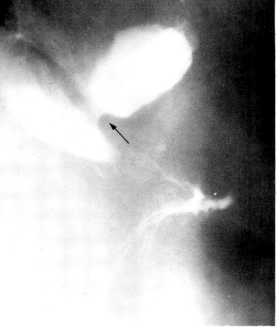

96 Oesophageal perforation. This chest x-ray shows subcutaneous emphysema in the neck and mediastinal emphysema due to oesophageal perforation following an upper gastrointestinal endoscopy. Perforation is usually traumatic (due to chest injuries, or ingestion of foreign bodies or caustic fluid). Oesophageal perforation is more common after rigid oesophagoscopy than after fibreoptic endoscopy. Oesophageal dilatation or prosthetic tube insertion may lead to perforation. Spontaneous perforation occurs rarely, for example due to violent vomiting.

97 Oesophageal perforation. A barium swallow performed one week after instrumental perforation of the oesophagus—outlining a large abscess cavity in the mediastinum, draining into the oesophagus and stomach. Surgical closure of oesophageal perforation is not always necessary—many patients respond to conservative management using parenteral feeding and broad spectrum antibiotics.

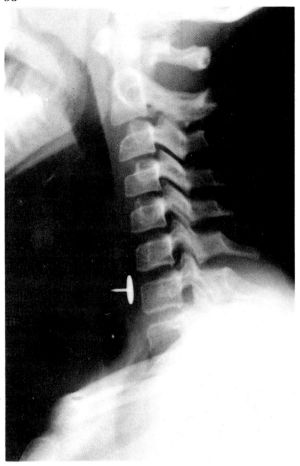

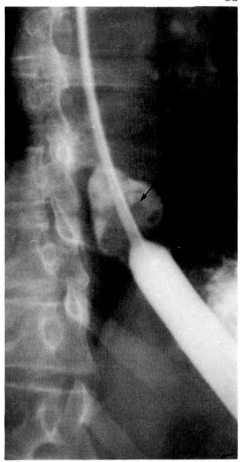

98   Oesophageal foreign body. This lateral
cervical radiograph shows a drawing pin impacted
in the cricopharyngeal region. Oesophageal foreign
bodies are most common in children, the mentally
handicapped and the elderly. Foreign bodies may
be removed endoscopically, using a snare or
grasping forceps passed down the biopsy channel
of the instrument.

99   Oesophageal foreign body. This x-
ray shows a piece of chicken impacted in
the lower oesophagus. In the absence of
oesophageal disease most objects impact
in the lower oesophagus, although
impaction in the mid-oesophagus can
occur. In this patient a contrast-filled
balloon was used to push the food bolus
into the stomach under radiological
control (it is more usual to remove such
an object by grasping it under
endoscopic direct vision).

CHAPTER 4

The Normal Stomach and Duodenum

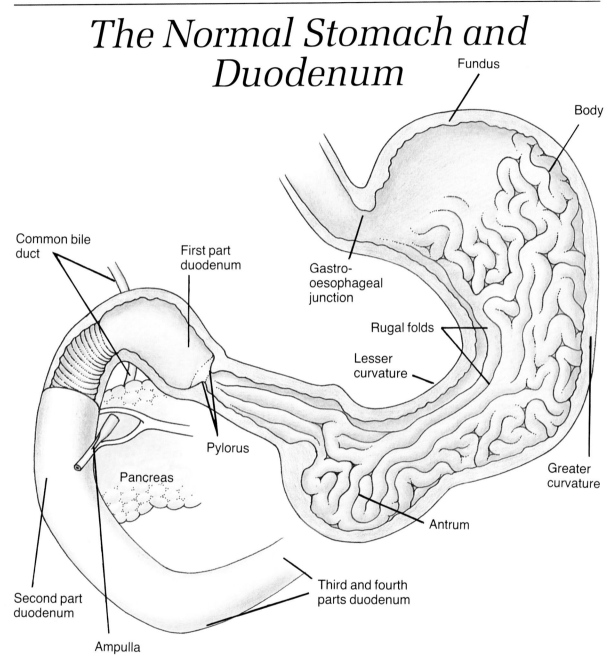

The stomach acts as a reservoir for food, and secretes acid to aid peptic digestion; intragastric acidity also sterilises the gastric contents, thereby decreasing any hazard from orally-ingested enteric pathogens. Emptying occurs periodically via the pyloric canal. The stomach is lined by mucus-secreting columnar epithelium. Beneath the submucosa lie three smooth muscle layers—the inner oblique, middle circular and outer longitudinal layers. The circular fibres are present everywhere except at the fundus, and they are greatly increased at the pylorus where they form a sphincter. The striking feature on gross inspection of the opened or empty stomach is the presence of rugal folds, which lie longitudinally, aiding the passage of solids and liquids towards the gastric antrum.

The blood supply to the stomach is derived from the coeliac axis. The right and left gastric arteries form an arch close to the lesser curvature. The right and left gastro-epiploic arteries form an arch some distance away from the greater curvature. Short gastric arteries arise from the splenic artery, and these supply the gastric fundus. Venous drainage is into the portal system, unless portal hypertension is present when venous blood may flow via the left gastric vein, through oesophageal varices and into the azygos system. The autonomic nervous system supplies sympathetic fibres (via the coeliac plexus) and parasympathetic fibres (arising from branches of the anterior and posterior vagal trunks).

The first part of the duodenum is only a few centimetres long. Its mucous membrane is smooth but the rest of the duodenum contains transverse folds, called valvuli conniventes. The ampulla of Vater is a tiny orifice situated on the medial wall of the second part of the duodenum. The common bile duct and pancreatic duct form a common opening at the ampulla of Vater, allowing flow of pancreatic juice and bile into the duodenum. This flow is regulated to some extent by the sphincter of Oddi, which encircles the ampulla. The blood supply to the head of the pancreas and duodenum derives from the superior and inferior pancreatico-duodenal arteries.

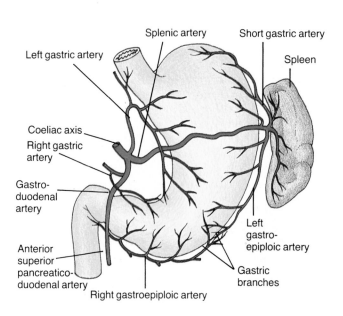

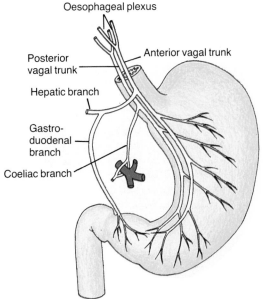

Arterial supply to the stomach. A diagram to show the arteries that arise from the coeliac axis to supply the stomach, duodenum, head of pancreas and spleen. The short gastric arteries arise from the splenic artery to supply the gastric fundus. The lesser curvature receives blood from branches of the left gastric artery, and the left and right gastroepiploic arteries perfuse the greater curvature. The antrum, pylorus and first part of duodenum are supplied by the gastroduodenal artery.

Vagal innervation. Parasympathetic nerve fibres from the anterior and posterior vagal trunks modulate gastric secretion and motility. The gastroduodenal branch of the anterior vagus plays an important role in gastric emptying. Surgical approaches to benign peptic ulcer include division of the vagal trunks or selective interruption of their branches.

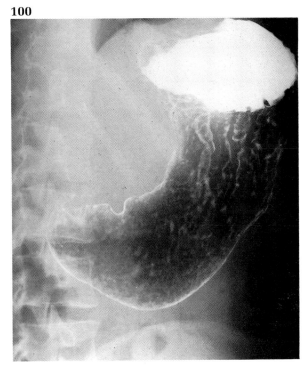

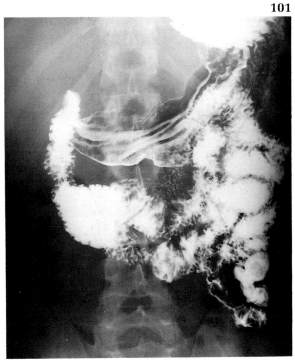

100 **Normal barium meal.** This double-contrast barium radiograph demonstrates the rugae of the gastric body and the smoother antral lining. This double-contrast appearance is achieved by taking a radiograph with the patient recumbent after swallowing barium and a bicarbonate–citric acid mixture.

101 **Normal barium meal.** The same study as **100**. Barium has now flowed into the duodenum and upper jejunum. The normal feathery mucosal appearance of the small intestine is shown.

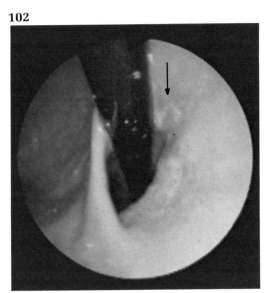

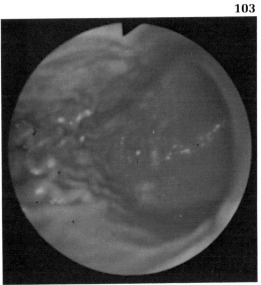

102 **The oesophago-gastric junction,** seen from below after inversion of the tip of the fibreoptic endoscope. The junction between the pink squamous oesophageal epithelium and the orange gastric columnar epithelium is arrowed.

103 **Normal body of stomach,** seen on endoscopy. The stomach has been filled with air, showing the rugae of the gastric body.

104

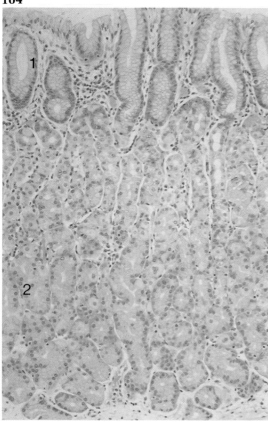

104   Normal body of stomach. The superficial epithelium consists of foveolar cells (1). The lower three-quarters of the epithelium (2) consists of specialised glands with acid-producing parietal cells (oxyntic) and zymogenic chief cells. The close packing of the glands in the normal stomach body leaves little space for connective tissue, and the inflammatory cell population of the lamina propria is normally minimal.

105   Normal stomach. Gastric mucosa at the transformation zone, where the gastric body type epithelium with its specialised glands (1) changes into gastric antral type epithelium with 'non-specialised' glands (2).

106   Normal stomach. The same field as in **105** stained with a combined stain for acid and neutral mucins, alcian blue–diastase PAS. The antral-type glands and the superficial epithelium stain red, reflecting their content of neutral mucins, whereas the deeper part of the specialised glands on the lower right are unstained since they have other secretory products.

105

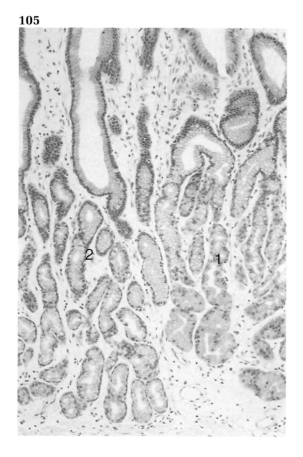

106

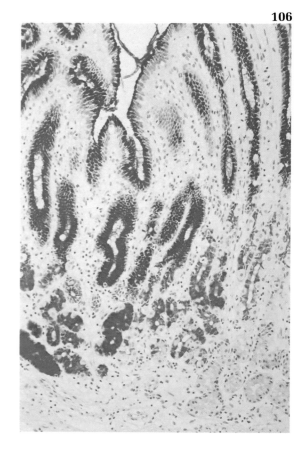

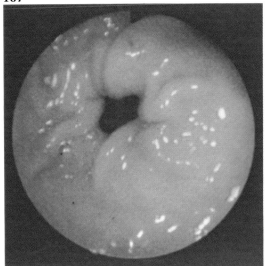

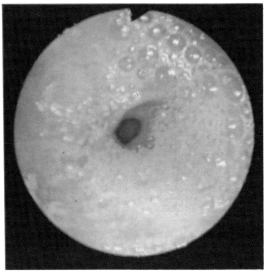

107 Normal pylorus. The pylorus is beginning to contract. Spasm of the pylorus may occasionally hinder intubation of the duodenum with the endoscope.

108 Bile reflux. Duodeno-gastric reflux of bile has occurred through the pylorus. Reflux of duodenal fluid containing bile and pancreatic secretions may occur in normal individuals, but it may be increased in patients with gastric ulceration. Major duodeno-gastric reflux occurs when the distal antrum and pylorus are resected or bypassed, as in Billroth I gastrectomy or gastroenterostomy.

109

109 Mucosa and submucosa of the gastric antrum. A heaped fold of normal mucosa is seen with a furrow (areae gastricae) on each side.

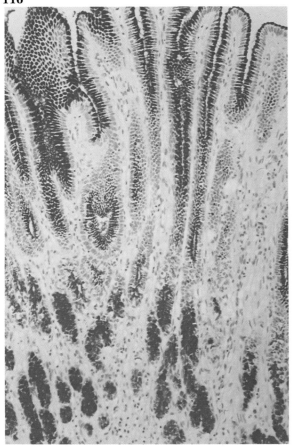

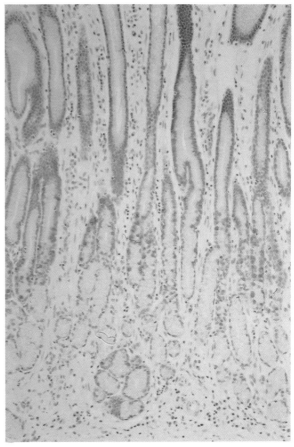

110   Normal gastric antrum. An alcian blue–diastase PAS stain for mucin shows the normal neutral mucin expression of the gastric antrum.

111   Normal gastric antrum. An immunoperoxidase stain for gastrin in the gastric antral mucosa. The normal number of brown-staining gastrin cells ('G-cells') are seen in the glandular epithelium.

112

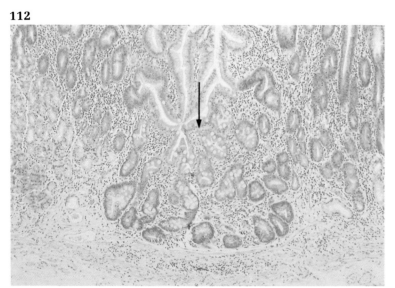

112   Chronically inflamed gastric antral mucosa. As well as a notable increase in the inflammatory cell population, the character of the epithelium has changed completely. In the centre of the field there is a focus of complete intestinal metaplasia (arrow), identified histologically by the clear round spaces representing goblet cells, and red-staining Paneth cells seen in the crypts.

113 Chronically inflamed gastric body mucosa, stained with alcian blue–diastase PAS. The single gland in the middle has changed from a specialised gastric body gland (1) and now resembles a large intestinal gland, and the red-staining neutral mucin of the normal stomach is altered to the bluish purple colour of the acid mucus normally secreted by the goblet cells of the large intestine. A normal gastric body gland is shown on the lower left of the field for comparison (2).

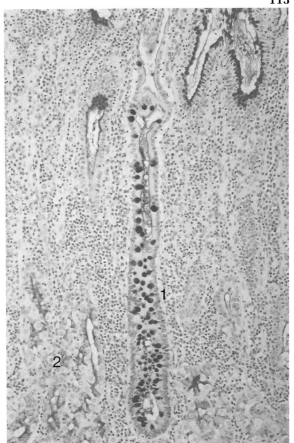

114 Normal duodenum. This hypotonic double-contrast duodenogram demonstrates the radiological appearance of the duodenal mucosa. To achieve this appearance the stomach and duodenum are distended by the administration of gas-releasing tablets or granules, or by asking the patient to swallow a drink with a high carbon dioxide content. The characteristic circular folds of the small intestine, the valvulae conniventes, are seen.

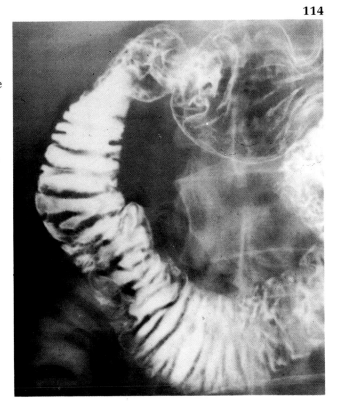

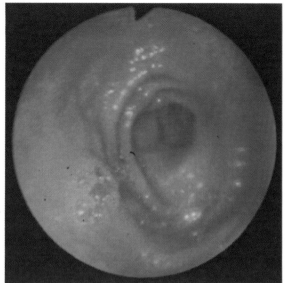

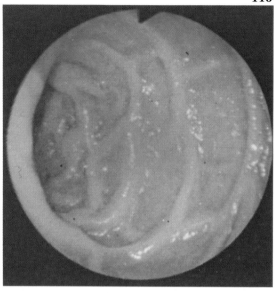

115   Normal duodenal bulb. This endoscopic view of the first part of the duodenum shows the smooth mucosal appearance. This is the most common site for peptic ulceration.

116   Normal second part of duodenum. The circular valvulae conniventes of this region are seen in this endoscopic photograph.

117

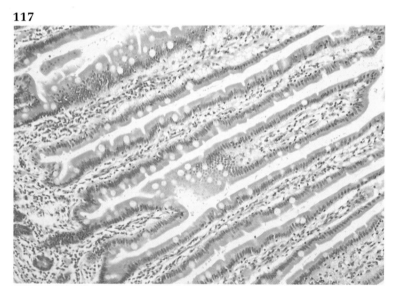

117   Normal duodenum. The long, thin, finger-like villi of the normal duodenal mucosa are seen in this photomicrograph.

118

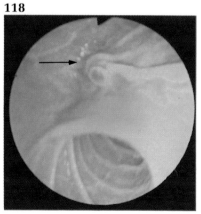

118   Papilla of Vater, shown by means of a side-viewing endoscope before retrograde cholangiopancreatography (arrow). Bile can be seen draining into the second part of the duodenum. The endoscopic appearance and position of the ampulla is variable, but it is usually present above a longitudinal fold. In this case two tiny longitudinal folds can be seen lying beneath the ampulla.

CHAPTER 5
Diseases of the Stomach and Duodenum

119

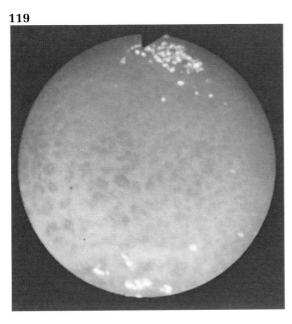

120

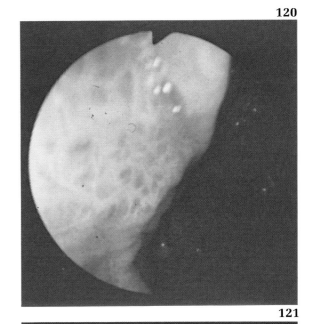

121

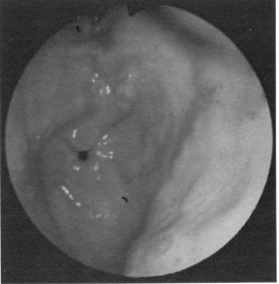

119 to **121** **Gastritis.** These three endoscopic views demonstrate some of the varied mucosal appearances seen in gastritis. These may range from superficial punctate areas of erythema in **119** to the frankly haemorrhagic areas of gastritis seen in the pre-pyloric region in **121**. The relationship between gastritis and peptic ulceration remains poorly understood. Gastric mucosal injury from a variety of agents (for example, alcohol and non-steroidal anti-inflammatory drugs) may produce similar appearances. It is now known that the bacterium *Campylobacter pylori* is frequently found in areas of gastritis, and may be important in its pathogenesis.

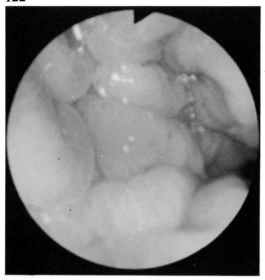

122 Congestive gastropathy. This endoscopic view of the body of the stomach shows congestive oedematous folds in a patient with portal hypertension. This appearance probably results from congestion of gastric venules.

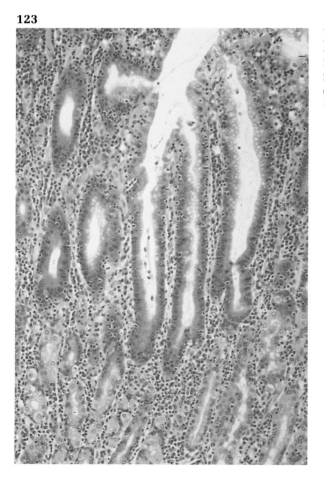

123 Gastritis. A photomicrograph of the histological appearances of chronically inflamed gastric body mucosa. It is now recognised that this histological appearance can result from the presence of *Campylobacter pylori* in the stomach.

124 Gastritis. At high magnification bacteria are seen within the surface mucus and adherent to the surface of the foveolar cells (arrow). The slightly curved rod-shaped organisms display the morphological characteristics of *Campylobacter pylori.*

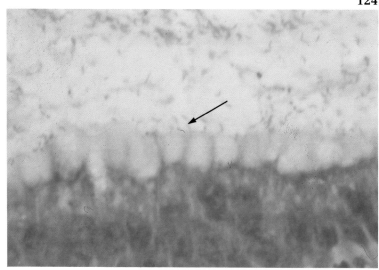

125 Gastritis. Silver staining (Warthin–Starry) identifies these *Campylobacter pylori* more clearly.

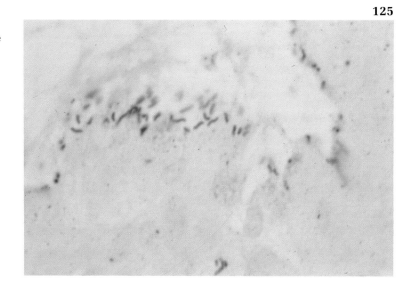

126 *Campylobacter pylori.* A scanning electron micrograph of rod-shaped Campylobacters lying on the gastric mucosal surface.

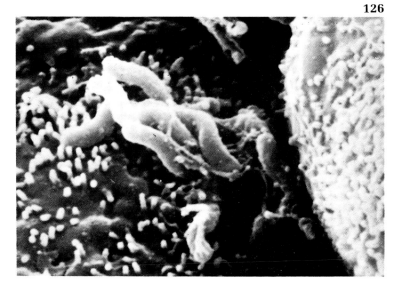

127

128

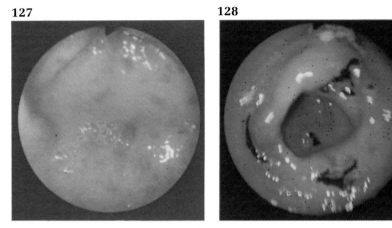

127 and **128 Gastric erosions.** These endoscopic views demonstrate superficial erosions of the antral mucosa in two patients who had been taking non-steroidal anti-inflammatory drugs. Other agents that may cause gastric mucosal injury include alcohol and corrosives. Similar erosions may be seen in patients with critical illnesses such as extensive burns. These lesions may be asymptomatic or may present with dyspepsia or gastrointestinal haemorrhage. The endoscopic appearances range from tiny superficial areas of erythema or ulceration (**127**) to confluent areas of ulceration (**128**). Double-contrast barium radiology may miss these superficial erosions, and endoscopy is required for diagnosis.

129

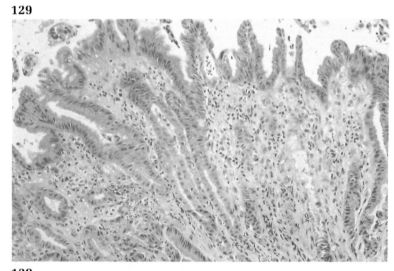

129 Gastric mucosal injury. An inflamed regenerative gastric antral mucosa. In this case the inflammation was due to a non-steroidal anti-inflammatory drug given for rheumatoid arthritis. The epithelium, which is attempting to heal, shows alarming reactive changes which could be mistaken for dysplasia.

130

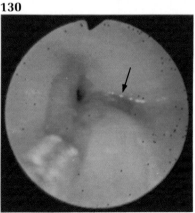

130 Mallory–Weiss tear, seen on endoscopic examination of the oesophago-gastric junction. A linear mucosal tear is arrowed. The Mallory–Weiss syndrome is now recognised as a common cause of acute upper gastrointestinal bleeding. The syndrome was originally described in alcoholics who had developed haematemesis after severe bouts of vomiting following heavy drinking.

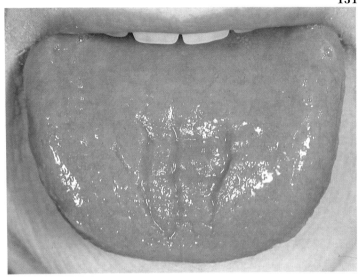

131 Pernicious anaemia. This disorder occurs as a result of autoimmune destruction of gastric parietal cells, leading to reduction of intrinsic factor secretion and consequent failure to absorb vitamin B_{12}. Patients with this disorder also fail to secrete acid into the stomach. This photograph shows a reddened, inflamed and fissured tongue (the so-called raw beef tongue) in a patient with vitamin B_{12} deficiency due to pernicious anaemia.

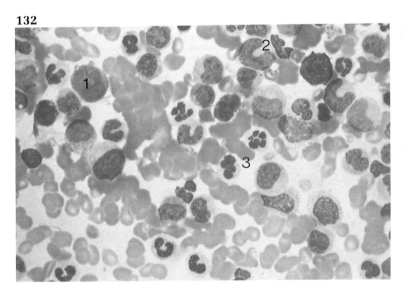

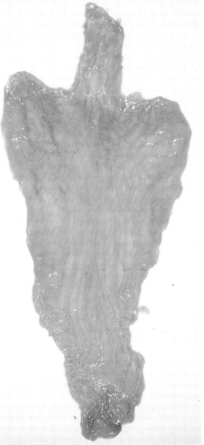

132 Pernicious anaemia. This bone marrow aspirate shows the characteristic megaloblastic changes. The bone marrow is hypercellular and the myeloid:erythroid ratio is reduced. The developing red cells are larger than normal and show a primitive nuclear chromatin (1), despite normal maturation and haemoglobinisation of the cytoplasm. Large abnormally shaped metamyelocytes (2) and megakaryocytes with hypersegmented nuclear lobes (3) are often present. The severity of these changes reflect the degree of anaemia.

133 Pernicious anaemia. The loss of gastric folds and pale atrophic mucosa are particularly prominent in the body of this stomach.

134

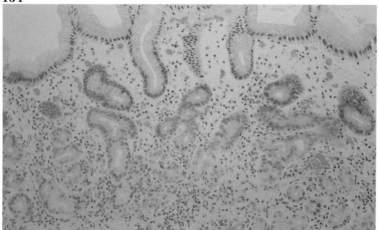

134 Pernicious anaemia. The mucosa of the gastric body in a patient with pernicious anaemia. The specialised glands have been replaced by antral-type glands which can be shown by immunohistochemistry to contain gastrin cells (normally only found in the antrum). This is part of the generalised, probably reactive, increase in gastrin cells in this condition. The lamina propria shows an increase in chronic inflammatory cells.

135

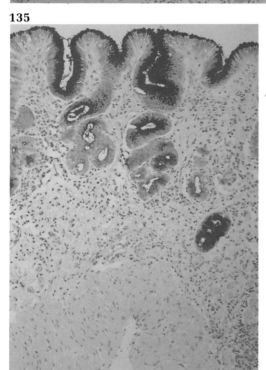

135 Pernicious anaemia. The thinned mucosa of the gastric body of a patient with pernicious anaemia, stained with alcian blue–diastase PAS to illustrate the neutral mucinous content of the glands in this area of pyloric metaplasia.

136

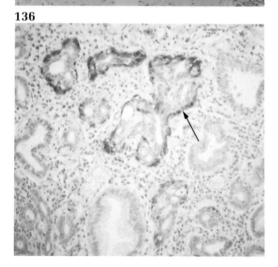

136 Pernicious anaemia. A biopsy of the gastric body from a patient with pernicious anaemia, stained by an immunoperoxidase technique for PGP 9.5, a neuroendocrine marker. A sleeve-like, periglandular proliferation of endocrine cells is seen (arrow).

137   Gastric carcinoid tumours.
The body of the stomach of a patient
with multiple small mucosal
carcinoid tumours, seen as scattered
round nodules (arrows). These
tumours are occasionally seen in the
gastric body in patients with
pernicious anaemia. However, this
example does not show the atrophic
mucosa usually seen in that
condition. Gastric carcinoids are
usually benign and have a good
prognosis, unlike carcinoids arising
elsewhere in the gut (see **346** to **350**).

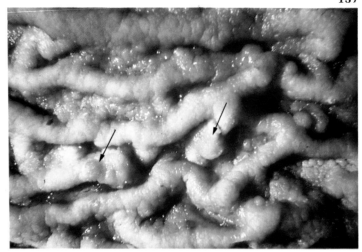

137

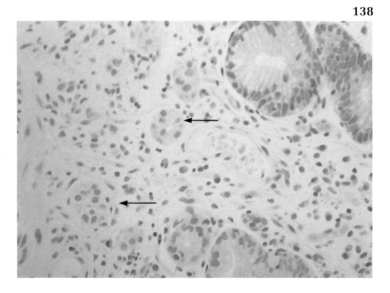

138

138   Gastric carcinoid tumours.
These scattered endocrine
hyperplasias may be inconspicuous
on microscopy. In this patient with
pernicious anaemia, scattered nests
of endocrine cells (arrows)
representing 'micro-carcinoids' are
seen between the gland bases and
the muscularis mucosa to the left.
It is believed that the proliferation of
these enterochromaffin-like cells is
due to hypergastrinaemia, which in
turn is due to achlorhydria.

139   Benign gastric ulcer. A small lesser curve gastric
ulcer is seen at the top of this endoscopic photograph (1).
Part of a larger benign ulcer crater is seen on the right (2).
Gastric ulcers usually present with dyspepsia or
epigastric pain, or with a complication such as
haemorrhage or perforation. The pathogenesis of gastric
ulceration is poorly understood: it is probably
multifactorial, involving gastric acid and pepsin
production, impaired mucosal resistance and the vascular
supply to the gastric mucosa. Non-steroidal anti-
inflammatory drugs are strongly associated with
perforation and haemorrhage from gastric and duodenal
ulcers, but it is not certain whether these agents actually
cause ulcers or complicate pre-existing ones.

139

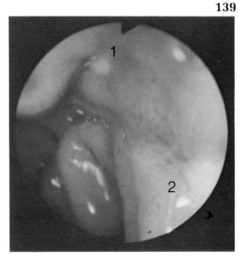

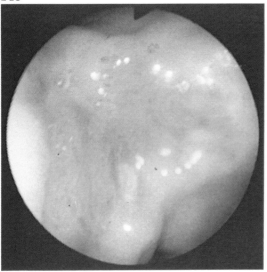

140 **Benign gastric ulcer.** This endoscopic view shows an ulcer surrounded by distortion of the surrounding mucosa at the angulus of the stomach.

141 **Benign gastric ulcer.** Endoscopic brush cytology is being undertaken on the gastric ulcer here to exclude malignancy. It is important to perform brush cytology and endoscopic biopsy of all gastric ulcers, because malignant ulcers may have the endoscopic appearance of benign ulcers. Gastric lymphomas can also produce a similar appearance. Endoscopic re-evaluation of gastric ulcer after 2 months of medical treatment is required to confirm ulcer healing.

142

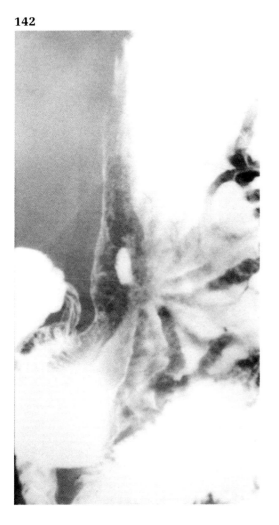

142 **Benign gastric ulcer.** This barium meal shows a deep lesser curve ulcer crater with surrounding folds of mucosa running towards the niche of barium within the ulcer crater.

143 Benign gastric ulcer. This large lesser curve gastric ulcer was found behind a fold. High lesser curve ulcers can easily be missed on endoscopy if inversion of the endoscope is not performed routinely to examine this region.

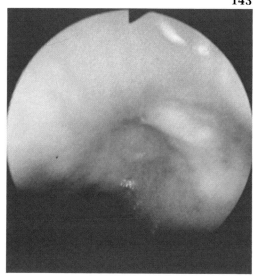

144 Benign gastric ulcer. This specimen was obtained from a patient who bled to death from the ulcer which had eroded an artery (seen in the base of the ulcer; arrow). The patient also had oesophageal varices.

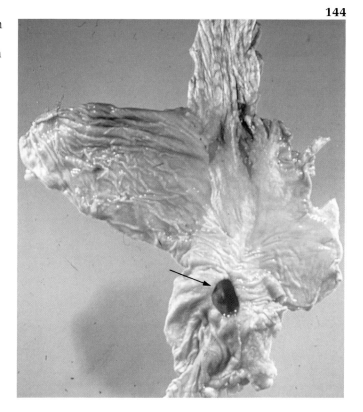

145

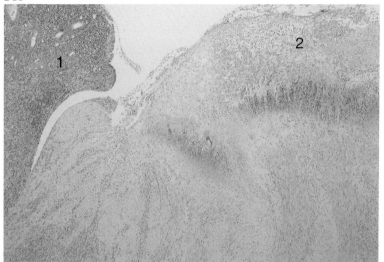

145   Benign gastric ulcer. The mucosa at the ulcer edge shows chronic inflammation (1). The ulcer base, seen on the right, consists of slough above (2), and inflamed fibrous connective tissue below. The pink-staining material seen at the lower right is a longitudinal section of a large artery in the ulcer base.

146

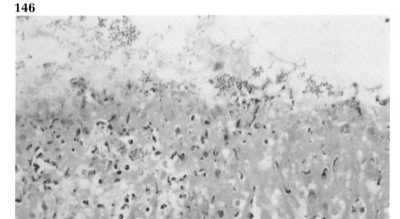

146   Benign gastric ulcer. The inflammatory slough of the ulcer seen at high power includes superficial colonies of *Candida.*

147

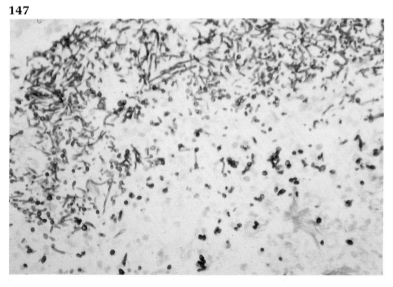

147   Benign gastric ulcer. The ulcer slough has been stained with the Grocott silver stain, which identifies the fungal hyphae of *Candida* in black. *Candida albicans* is found frequently in the slough of benign gastric ulcers, but its significance is uncertain.

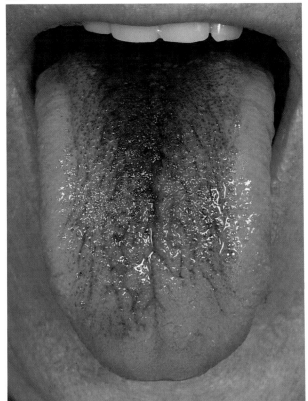

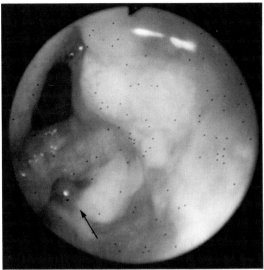

149 Haemorrhage from peptic ulcer. This endoscopic view of a pyloric ulcer demonstrates a vessel protruding (arrow) from within the ulcer slough of a patient who had recently suffered a major haematemesis. Re-bleeding commonly occurs from ulcers with visible vessels.

148 Bismuth staining of the tongue. Medical treatment of peptic ulcer includes the use of either the histamine H_2-receptor antagonists, sucralfate or tripotassium dicitrato-bismuthate. Tablets of the latter drug may have to be chewed before swallowing, and discoloration of the tongue may result.

150 Bleeding gastric ulcer, seen on emergency endoscopy in a patient with haematemesis and melaena. Urgent surgical treatment is usually necessary for patients who have arterial spurting from peptic ulcers. Endoscopic laser photocoagulation and heater probes are becoming more widely used for treating bleeding peptic ulcers or those with visible vessels.

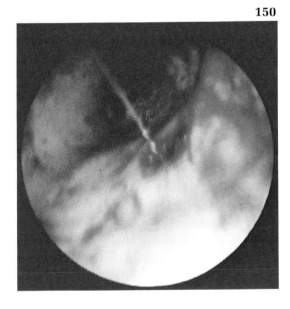

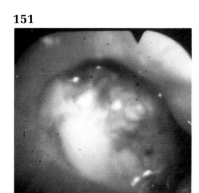

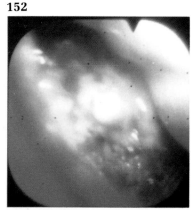

151 Endoscopic signs of recent haemorrhage in peptic ulcer. A 'visible vessel' is seen within the ulcer crater.

152 Post-laser photocoagulation. This shows the results of laser photocoagulation to the visible vessel identified in **151**, with obliterations of the vessel.

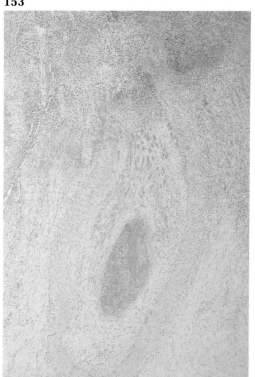

153 Benign gastric ulcer. The eroded artery on the floor of the ulcer shows endarteritis obliterans.

154 Gastric polyps. This post-mortem gastrectomy specimen shows multiple sessile and pedunculated adenomatous polyps. These may occur in isolation or be associated with familial polyposis syndromes. Malignant transformation may occur in up to 40% of true adenomatous polyps. Small hyperplastic polyps of the stomach are more common and have no significant cancer potential. Endoscopic snare diathermy excision is replacing the more aggressive policy of partial or total gastric resection. Regular endoscopic surveillance of such patients is necessary to diagnose and treat recurrent polyps and to screen for malignancy in this high-risk group.

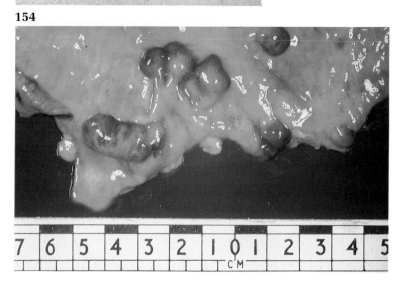

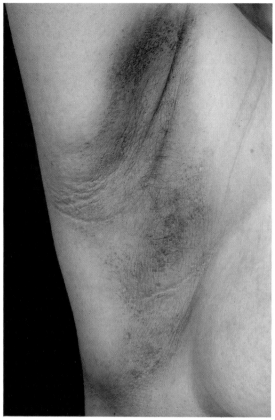

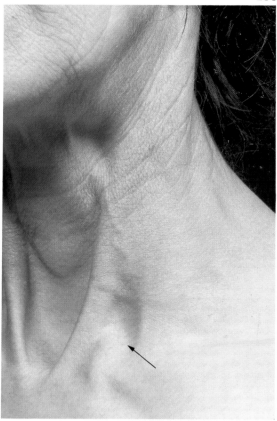

155   Acanthosis nigricans is a pigmentation and wartiness of the axilla and groins. The angles of the mouth and hands may also be involved. Patients with this disorder are commonly found to have underlying malignant disease (most commonly gastric, pancreatic or bronchial carcinoma).

156   Virchow's node. Left-sided supraclavicular lymphadenopathy (arrow) may be a sign of metastasis from intra-abdominal malignancy, particularly a gastric or pancreatic carcinoma.

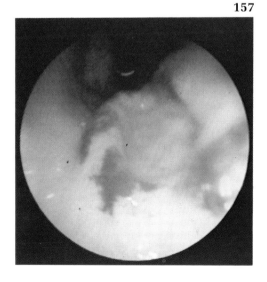

157   Gastric carcinoma. A large, malignant, lesser curve gastric ulcer is seen on inversion of the fibreoptic endoscope. Endoscopic features suggesting malignancy include the raised rolled ulcer margins and irregular surrounding mucosal folds. Brush cytology (**141**) and multiple endoscopic biopsies (**163**) are required to exclude malignancy in all patients with gastric ulcers.

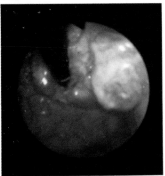

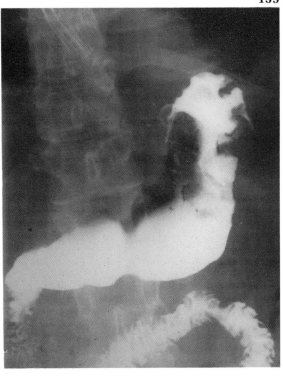

158   Gastric carcinoma. This polypoid carcinoma of the gastric fundus was also identified by inversion of the fibreoptic endoscope. This particular carcinoma had spread submucosally into the lower oesophagus, and the patient presented with dysphagia.

159   Gastric carcinoma. This barium meal identified a large polypoid carcinoma of the lesser curve of the stomach (the patient had no history of dyspepsia, but presented with spinal metastases).

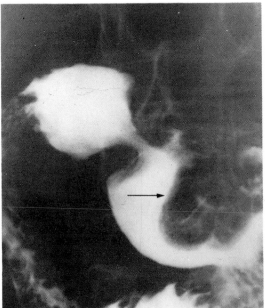

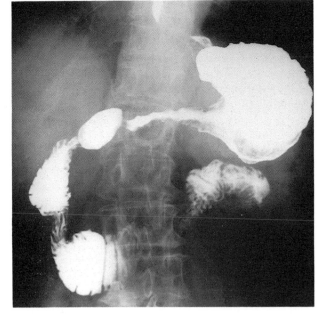

160   Gastric carcinoma. Barium meal demonstrating a polypoid carcinoma of the antrum (arrow), which had caused recurrent bouts of vomiting due to periodic blockade of the pylorus.

161   Linitis plastica of the stomach. This barium meal demonstrates diffuse involvement of the body and antrum of the stomach by linitis plastica, a form of gastric carcinoma that infiltrates the gastric submucosa. Sometimes the whole stomach is involved with this form of carcinoma, which carries a very poor prognosis.

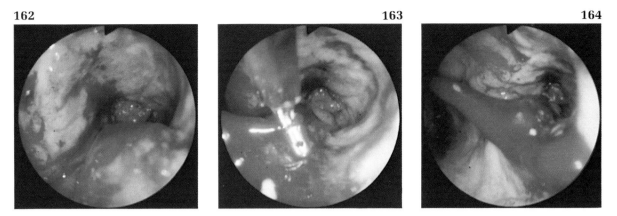

162 to 164   **Linitis plastica of the stomach. 162** shows the mucosa encased by adenocarcinoma. **163** shows endoscopic biopsy of the lesion, which has resulted in brief haemorrhage **164.**

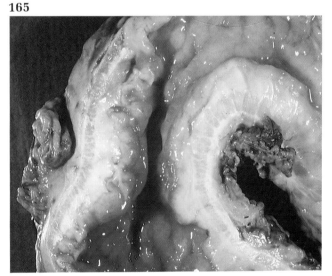

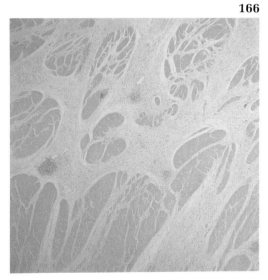

165   **Linitis plastica.** This post-mortem appearance demonstrates the submucosal infiltration of the stomach wall by the pale tumour tissue. The mucosa is congested but does not show the mucosal irregularity of a carcinoma.

166   **Linitis plastica.** The darkly pink-staining muscle bundles are diffusely infiltrated by poorly differentiated carcinoma of linitis plastica type. The blue-staining islands are areas of chronic inflammation, the pale pink is the fibrous tissue reaction which often accompanies this type of carcinoma (the individual carcinoma cells are not visible at this magnification).

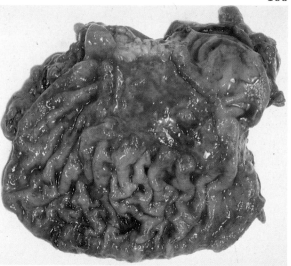

168 Gastric carcinoma. This surgical resection specimen demonstrates a large, malignant gastric ulcer with irregular surrounding folds and rolled edges. Blood clot is visible from recent haemorrhage from this ulcer.

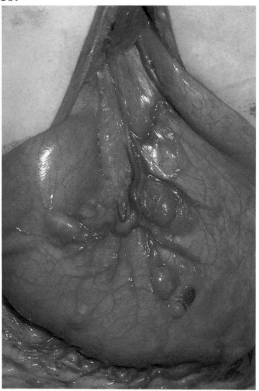

167 Gastric carcinoma. This operative photograph shows nodules of tumour tissue outside the lesser curve of the stomach. The prognosis of gastric carcinoma is poor when the tumour has penetrated the muscularis propria.

169

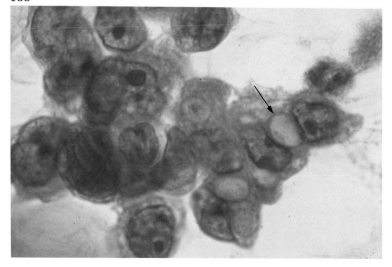

169 Gastric carcinoma. A gastric brushing stained with the Papanicolaou method. Pleomorphic malignant cells with prominent nucleoli and a clumped nuclear chromatin pattern are seen. A few of the cells show intracytoplasmic vacuoles, probably containing mucin (arrow).

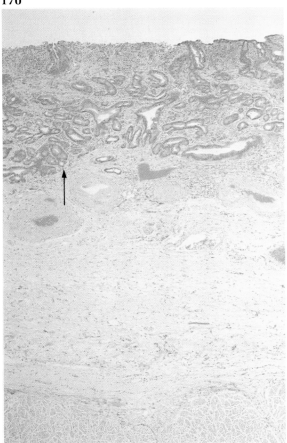

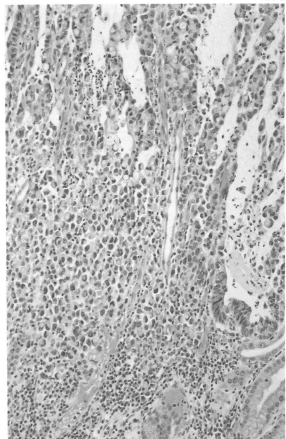

170 Early gastric carcinoma. A superficial gastric carcinoma (intestinal type) of the gastric cardia. Moderately differentiated neoplastic glands are seen infiltrating the upper part of the submucosa (arrow). Since the muscularis propria is not involved by tumour, this lesion qualifies as an early gastric carcinoma. Early gastric carcinomas carry a good prognosis following surgical removal. Unfortunately, most gastric carcinoma patients present with more advanced disease.

171 Gastric carcinoma. The mucosa of a patient with poorly differentiated, signet ring adenocarcinoma of the stomach. The epithelium on the lower right shows chronic inflammation. There is an abrupt change to the tumour occupying the rest of the field.

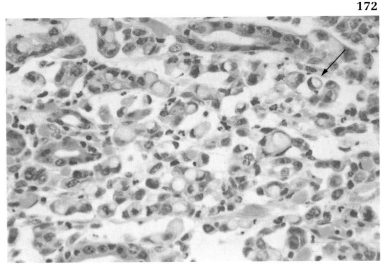

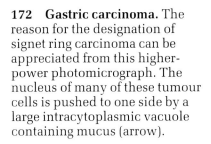

172 Gastric carcinoma. The reason for the designation of signet ring carcinoma can be appreciated from this higher-power photomicrograph. The nucleus of many of these tumour cells is pushed to one side by a large intracytoplasmic vacuole containing mucus (arrow).

173

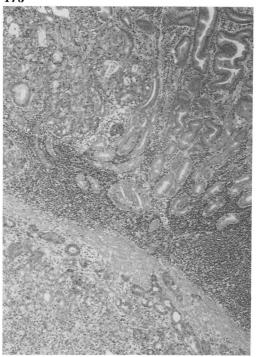

173 Gastric carcinoma. The edge of a moderately differentiated adenocarcinoma of intestinal type of the stomach. The epithelium on the right is inflamed, in the middle and left it is severely dysplastic, and infiltrative submucosal tumour is seen at the bottom.

174

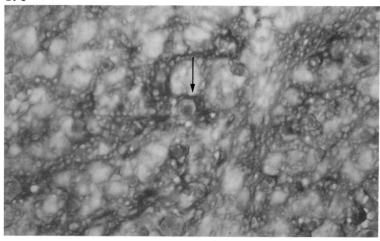

174 Gastric carcinoma. High-magnification photograph of a mucoid (colloid) carcinoma. This preparation is stained with alcian blue– diastase PAS, and the scanty tumour cells (pink) are seen in an ocean of acid mucus (arrow).

175

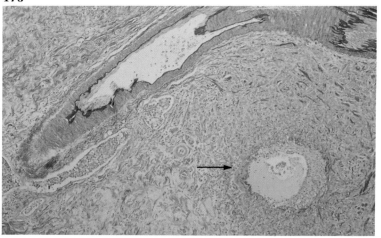

175 Gastric carcinoma. The submucosa of a patient with poorly differentiated adenocarcinoma of the stomach. In this preparation elastin is stained black and the collagen appears red. Beneath the artery, identified by its black elastic lamina, a cord of tumour cells is seen within lymphatic spaces on the left and diffusely infiltrating the wall of a vein, lower right (arrow).

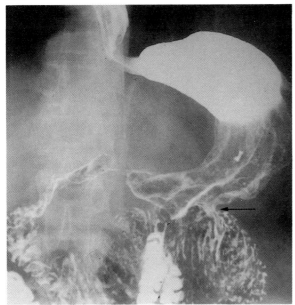

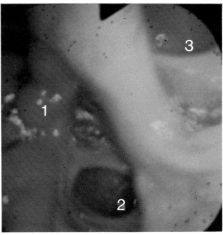

177 Gastro-enterostomy.
An endoscopic view of the
anastomosis between stomach and
jejunum. The reddened gastric
mucosa is seen on the left (1), the
efferent loop of the small intestine is
seen below (2), and the afferent loop
is on the upper right side (3).

176 Gastro-enterostomy. This double-contrast
barium meal shows flow of contrast from the
stomach through the stoma and into the jejunum
(arrow). A barium meal often helps in the
understanding of post-surgical anatomy, but an
endoscopy is also required for full assessment of
a post-surgical stomach.

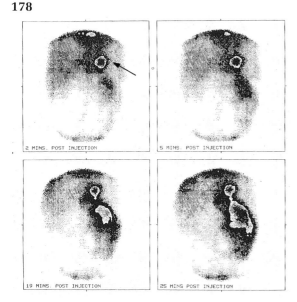

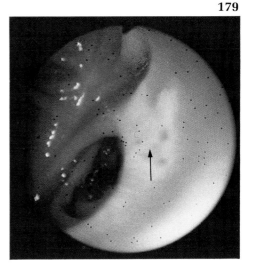

178 Gastric scan with technetium. Two
minutes after injection of technetium the isotope
accumulates in the gastric remnant (arrow). The
isotope then passes to the small intestine, via a
gastro-enterostomy. This test is used to identify
ectopic gastric mucosa—for example, after
gastric surgery or if a Meckel's diverticulum is
suspected (see **330**).

179 Stomal ulcer, seen on endoscopy
in a patient who had undergone a
Billroth II gastrectomy for Zollinger
Ellison syndrome. This patient
presented with iron deficiency
anaemia. The small brown areas of
blood clot within the ulcer slough
suggested that the patient had suffered
recent haemorrhage from the ulcer
(arrow).

180

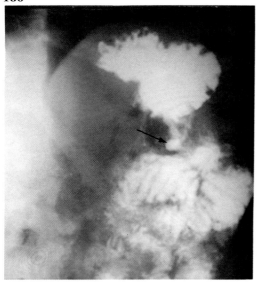

180 Stomal ulcer. This barium meal
shows an ulcer crater at the stoma (arrow).
Patients who have undergone partial
gastrectomy are at risk of developing
carcinoma 20 years or more after the
operation. Regular endoscopic
surveillance for early malignancy may be
indicated in patients who have undergone
partial gastrectomy for peptic ulcer 15
years or more previously, but this
screening policy has not been shown to be
cost-effective.

181 Carcinoma of gastric remnant. This surgical
resection shows a carcinoma that had developed at
the site of a previous partial gastrectomy with Billroth
II anastomosis.

182

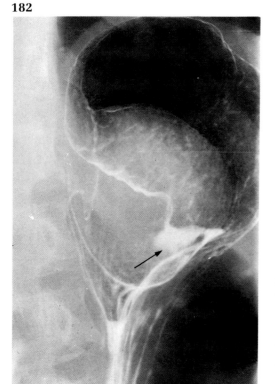

182 Gastric leiomyoma. This double-contrast barium
meal has demonstrated a huge smooth leiomyoma of
the lesser curve of the stomach with its characteristic
central ulcer crater (arrow). These are benign tumours
of the gastric smooth muscle. They may present with
gastrointestinal haemorrhage, iron deficiency anaemia
or vague non-specific symptoms. Surgical wedge
resection is usually indicated, particularly if
haemorrhage has occurred.

183　Gastric leiomyoma. Endoscopic view, demonstrating apical ulceration, which is the site of bleeding.

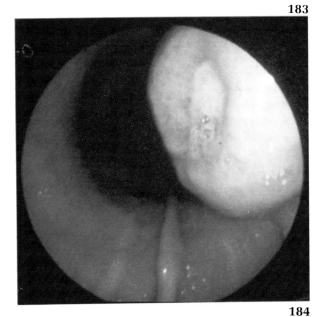

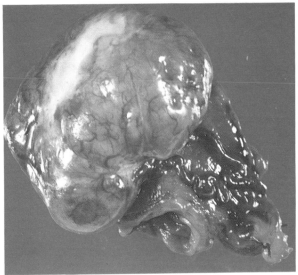

184　Gastric leiomyoma. This resection specimen has the smooth polypoid appearance of a leiomyoma and a linear ulcer crater on its summit. The ulcer may be due to pressure necrosis from the expanding submucosal tumour.

185　Gastric leiomyoma. Histological appearance of the rounded tumour mass covered by a thin rim of submucosa and mucosa, with central ulceration and cavitation.

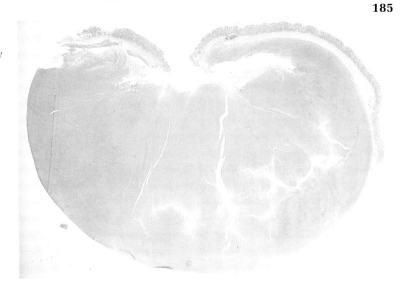

186

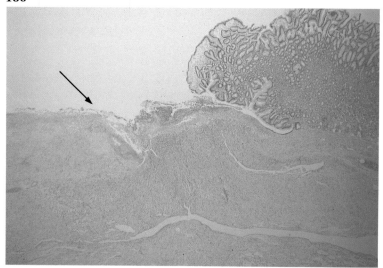

186 Gastric leiomyoblastoma.
Occasionally smooth muscle tumours of the stomach consist of cells with clear cytoplasm as here, rather than the pink staining of the more usual tumour. These are termed 'leiomyoblastomas' or 'Stout's peculiar tumour'. They commonly show overlying ulceration (arrow).

187

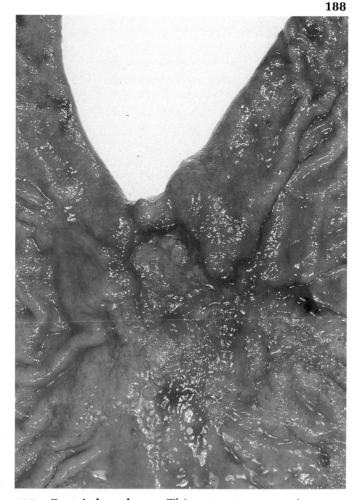

188

187 Gastric lymphoma.
An endoscopic view of a nodule of lymphoma tissue with superficial ulceration. The endoscopic appearances of gastric lymphomas may vary from multiple ulcerated nodules to giant infiltrated rugae. The tumours may arise submucosally, so that endoscopic biopsy is frequently negative. The stomach is the most frequent site for primary extranodal non-Hodgkin's lymphoma. Gastric involvement in a more generalised lymphomatous process may also occur. The clinical presentation of gastric lymphoma is similar to that of gastric carcinoma, but the differential diagnosis is most important because the five-year survival following surgical resection of gastric lymphoma is about 50%. Radiotherapy and chemotherapy are valuable in the management of intra-abdominal lymphoma deposits.

188 Gastric lymphoma. This gastrectomy specimen contains a lymphoma with central ulceration, and small polypoid areas of tumour and irregular folds surrounding the ulcer.

189 Gastric lymphoma. This gastrectomy specimen demonstrates more diffuse involvement of the gastric mucosa with lymphoma tissue. This particular tumour was resected from an 18-year-old woman who presented with vague epigastric pain and weight loss.

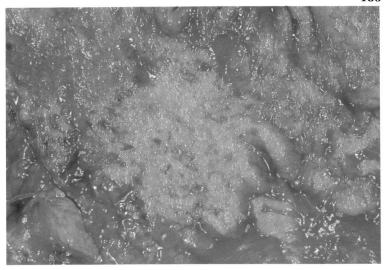

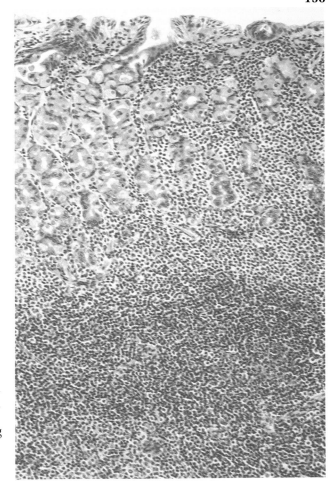

190 Gastric lymphomas are derived from mucosal associated lymphoid tissue. They often have an indolent course, remaining localised to their site of origin in the gut, and hence differ from nodal lymphomas in being amenable to surgical resection. Here the dark-staining lymphoma cells are infiltrating the gastric body mucosa in a diffuse fashion and have aggregated to form a follicle-like structure below.

191

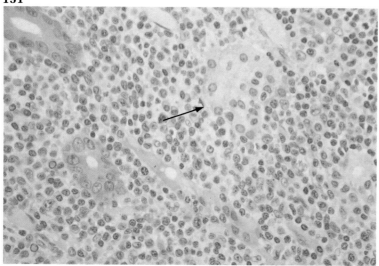

191　Gastric lymphoma.
At higher magnification this lymphoma is seen to consist of centrocyte-like cells which show a marked tendency to permeate the glandular epithelium (arrow).

192

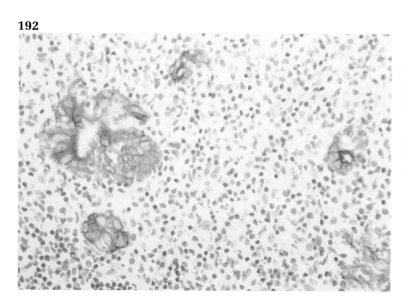

192　Gastric lymphoma.
Mucosal infiltration by neoplastic lymphocytes can lead to epithelial destruction. Here, immunostaining of the lymphoepithelial lesion for Cam 5.2 (a low molecular weight cytokeratin—a marker for the gastric epithelium) highlights the epithelial remnant in brown.

193

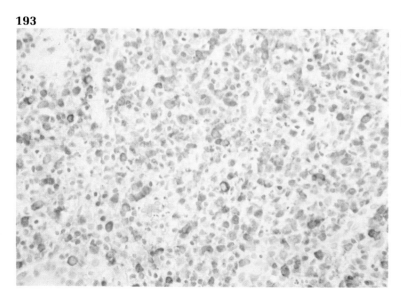

193　Gastric lymphoma. Many of these tumours have an IgM Kappa immunophenotype. This immunoperoxidase preparation shows the predominant expression of Kappa-light chains by this lymphoma.

194 Ménétrier's disease. A barium meal showing the giant gastric rugal hypertrophy. This disease commonly presents with ulcer-like dyspepsia or gastrointestinal haemorrhage from superimposed peptic ulceration or diffuse haemorrhagic gastritis. Some patients have weight loss and hypoproteinaemia with ascites or oedema.

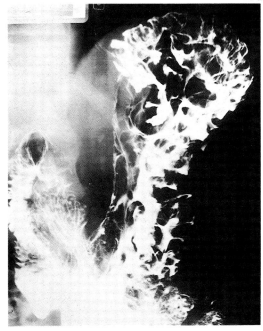

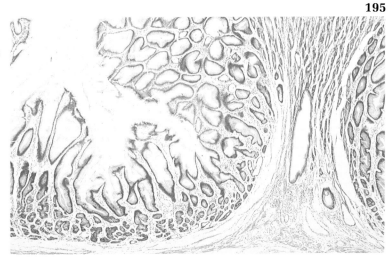

195 Ménétrier's disease. A photomicrograph showing marked hypertrophy of the gastric body mucosa with a raised giant ruga on the right. There is a dilated gland base within the pedicle of this fold.

196 Ménétrier's disease. The superficial parts of the hyperplastic rugae of Ménétrier's disease show an increase of the foveolar cell zone and an unusual 'corkscrew' architecture.

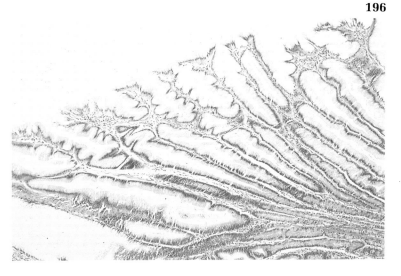

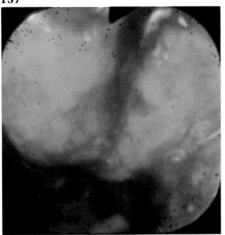

197 Chemical injury of oesophagus and stomach. This endoscopic view was obtained in a patient who had ingested hydrochloric acid. The oesophageal mucosa shows congestion, necrosis and inflammatory change. Severe damage may be present in the oesophagus and stomach in the absence of warning signs in the mouth or pharynx. Oesophageal stricture or perforation from the oesophagus or stomach, or from both, are possible complications. Gastric aspiration and lavage should be withheld for this reason; water or milk should be given by mouth. Cautious endoscopy may be indicated once the immediate emergency has passed.

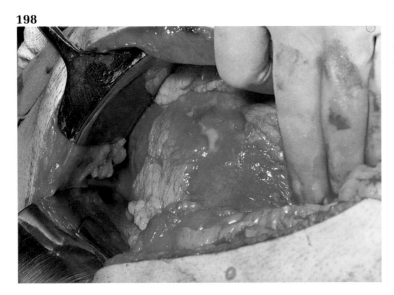

198 Chemical injuries of the oesophagus and stomach. This operative photograph was obtained from a patient who had developed signs of peritonitis following the ingestion of sodium hydroxide. An area of necrotic stomach can be seen in the centre of the photograph.

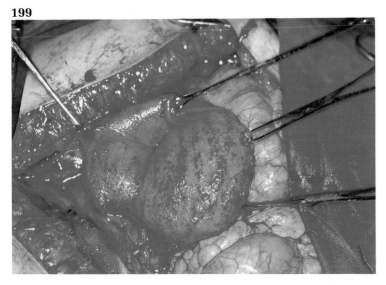

199 Vascular malformations of the stomach. An operative photograph showing the stomach opened, with submucous antral vascular malformations. These may present with gastrointestinal haemorrhage and the mucosal view obtained at endoscopy may miss the site of haemorrhage. Partial gastrectomy may be necessary to control the haemorrhage.

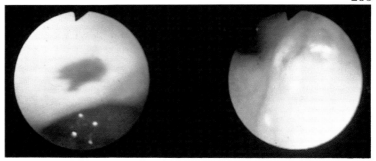

200   Vascular malformations of the stomach. Arterial vascular malformations or angiodysplastic areas can occur at any site in the gastrointestinal tract. The view on the left shows an arteriovenous malformation of the lesser curve of the stomach. This was treated by laser photocoagulation. The results of this may be seen in the photograph on the right. The malformation and surrounding mucosa have been blanched. Patients with multiple areas of angiodysplasia are well suited to laser therapy or heater probe treatment because the lesions may be treated individually as they occur.

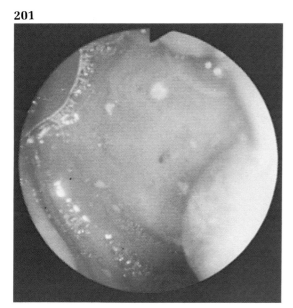

201   Duodenitis. An endoscopic view showing inflammation and multiple superficial erosions of duodenal mucosa giving rise to the so-called 'salt and pepper' appearance. Duodenitis commonly coexists with peptic ulceration of the duodenum or stomach. These changes are often found in the duodenal cap at endoscopy during investigation of patients with dyspepsia. Rarer causes of duodenitis include tuberculosis, Crohn's disease and viral infections.

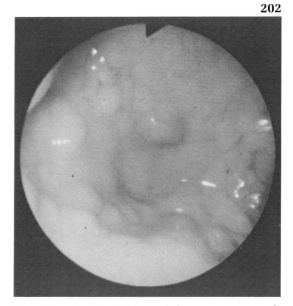

202   Duodenitis. This nodular appearance of the duodenal mucosa may follow recurrent episodes of duodenitis. Biopsy of the mucosa demonstrated acute and chronic inflammation.

203

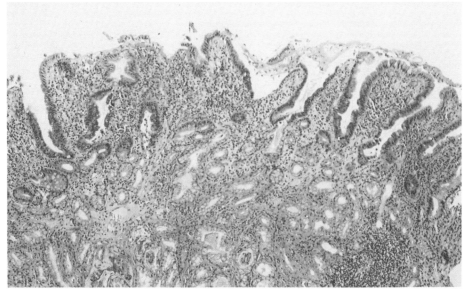

203 Duodenitis. A duodenal biopsy stained by the MSB technique. There is a superficial erosion and moderate inflammation.

204

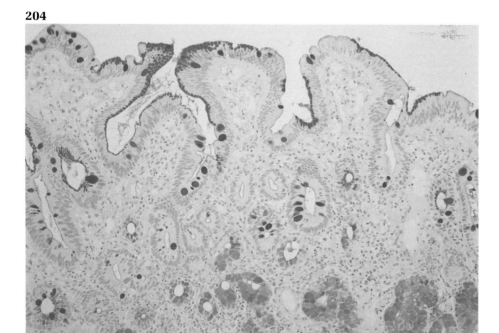

204 Duodenitis. At higher magnification and upon staining for alcian blue–diastase PAS it is clear that the normal blue-staining goblet cells of the duodenal villi have been replaced by superficial red-staining epithelium of gastric foveolar type. These changes, not unusual in duodenitis, may be associated with hypersecretion of acid by the stomach.

205 Duodenal ulcer. A double-contrast barium meal showing a small ulcer in the duodenal cap with mucosal folds radiating away from the ulcer crater (arrow). Endoscopy with biopsy is usually not required in patients who are found to have a duodenal ulcer on barium meal.

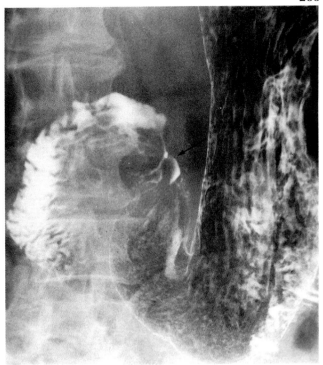

206 Duodenal ulcer, shown at endoscopy. The ulcer may occur in any part of the duodenal bulb. Less than 5% of duodenal ulcers occur beyond the first part of the duodenum; the presence of more distal ulcers raises the possibility of a gastrinoma.

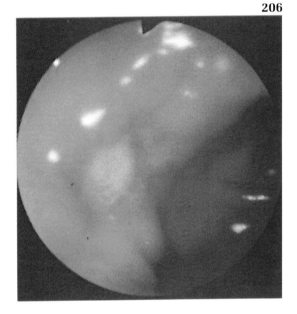

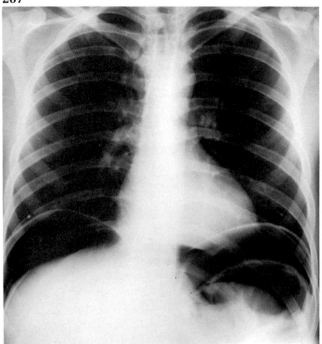

207 Perforated duodenal ulcer. This common emergency results in peritonitis and requires urgent surgical intervention. This chest x-ray confirms the presence of an intra-abdominal perforation that has produced gas under both hemi-diaphragms. The risk of perforation is increased in patients taking non-steroidal anti-inflammatory drugs.

208

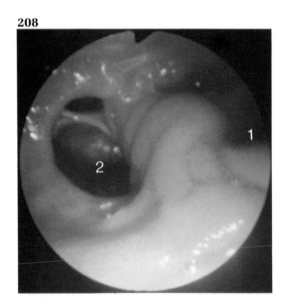

208 Peri-ampullary diverticulum. This endoscopic photograph of the papilla of Vater (containing the blue endoprosthesis, 1) also shows a peri-ampullary diverticulum (2). These diverticula are herniations of mucosa through the muscle coat of the bowel wall, and they may be present elsewhere in the small intestine. Endoscopic cannulation of the papilla may be difficult if it lies within or beside a peri-ampullary diverticulum.

209 Ampullary carcinoma. This barium meal shows a polypoid tumour arising from the peri-ampullary mucosa. Obstructive jaundice or pancreatic steatorrhoea, or both, occur early in the course of the disease. Other malignant tumours occasionally found in the duodenum include carcinoid, lymphoma and various sarcomata.

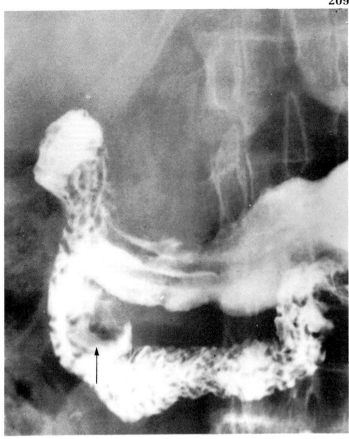

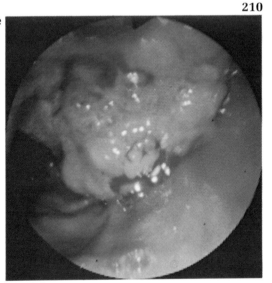

210 Ampullary carcinoma, shown at endoscopy to be growing into the duodenal lumen. Duodenal obstruction or haemorrhage are rare presenting features. This patient presented with the more common symptoms of obstructive jaundice and cholangitis. The endoscopist should confirm the diagnosis by biopsy.

211

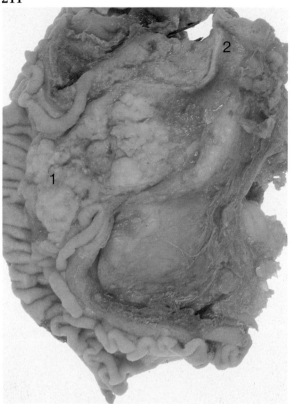

211 Ampullary carcinoma. A Whipple's pancreaticoduodenectomy has been performed. The pale tumour lies in the centre of the photograph (1), with the pancreas below it. The tumour is occluding the dilated common bile duct (2).

212

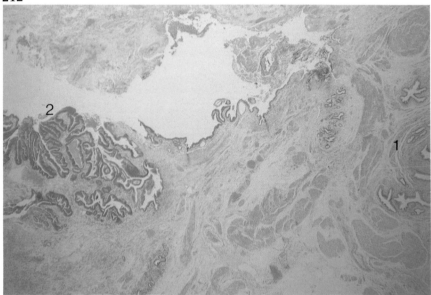

212 Ampullary carcinoma. A moderately differentiated adenocarcinoma of the ampulla of Vater. The pancreatic duct is seen on the right (1), tumour is seen on the left (2) and there is ulceration at the top.

CHAPTER 6

The Normal Pancreas and Pancreatic Disease

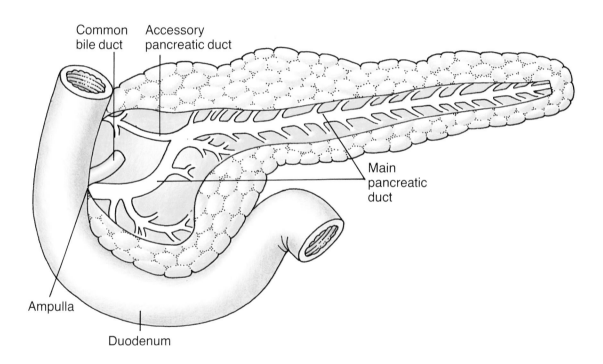

The pancreas lies retroperitoneally, in close relationship to the stomach, transverse colon and the second part of the duodenum, into which its main duct empties. It has two main functions: the production of exocrine secretion of enzymes and bicarbonate, which are important in digestion and the neutralisation of gastric acid, and the production of endocrine secretions (most importantly insulin) which drain into the portal venous blood and pass via the liver into the systemic circulation. A main and a separate accessory duct can be identified in most people. The main

pancreatic duct and common bile duct form a common terminal channel at the ampulla of Vater.

The head of the pancreas receives the bulk of its blood supply from the pancreatico-duodenal arteries. The rest of the gland is supplied by branches of the splenic artery. Venous drainage is into the portal system, mainly via branches of the splenic vein. Pancreatic secretion is stimulated by distension and the presence of acid in the second part of the duodenum; the stimulus is mediated by hormones such as cholecystokinin.

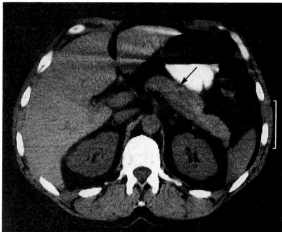

213   The normal pancreas. Computerised tomography is a major advance in the investigation of pancreatic disease. Here a normal body and tail of pancreas (arrow) are seen below the contrast-filled stomach.

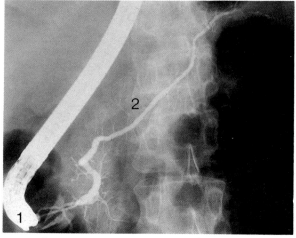

214   The normal pancreas at endoscopic retrograde pancreatography. A cannula has been inserted through a side-viewing endoscope (1) and manipulated into the pancreatic duct via the papilla. Injection of contrast medium has opacified the normal pancreatic duct and its side-branches (2).

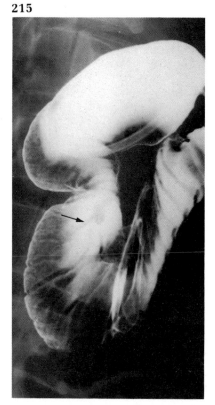

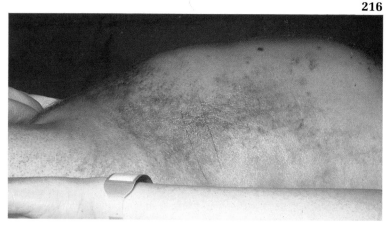

216   Acute pancreatitis. This patient with severe acute pancreatitis has developed jaundice and retroperitoneal haemorrhage following severe sudden epigastric pain and vomiting. The condition is diagnosed on the basis of the clinical picture and raised serum and urinary concentrations of pancreatic enzymes (amylase). In this patient the retroperitoneal haemorrhage from the necrotic pancreas has tracked into the left flank and produced ecchymotic discolouration (Grey–Turner's sign). Periumbilical bruising (Cullen's sign) may also be present.

215   Annular pancreas. The duodenal loop has been intubated and filled with air and barium. The papilla of Vater and its horizontal folds can just be seen beneath the constriction of the annular pancreas (arrow). This anatomical variant occurs when the ventral portion of the embryonic pancreas rotates incorrectly and encircles the second part of the duodenum. Patients may present with duodenal obstruction or acute pancreatitis.

217 Acute pancreatitis. The most common causes of acute pancreatitis are gallstones and alcohol excess. Less-common causes include accidental and operative trauma, hypercalcaemia, and drugs such as corticosteroids, azathioprine and diuretics. Hypertriglyceridaemia may also cause pancreatitis. Lipaemic serum (arrow) may be a clue to the presence of hypertriglyceridaemia, which may be familial or acquired as a result of alcohol excess. Lipaemic serum may conceal the elevation in serum amylase levels in pancreatitis complicating hypertriglyceridaemia.

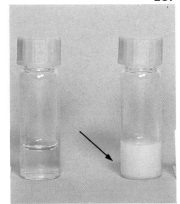

217

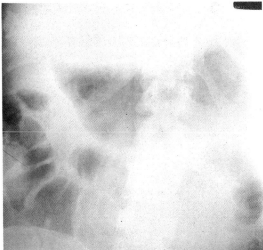

218

218 Acute pancreatitis. This plain abdominal x-ray shows gaseous distension of the stomach and small intestinal loops due to acute pancreatitis. The small intestinal loop on the right of the photograph is the so-called sentinel loop. The appearance of this x-ray is not specific for acute pancreatitis, and may be seen in ileus due to other causes.

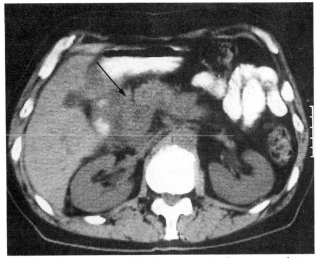

219

219 Acute pancreatitis. Computerised tomographic scanning has demonstrated a grossly swollen pancreas (arrow).

220 Acute pancreatitis. This post-mortem specimen was obtained from a patient who died from acute pancreatitis. The grossly haemorrhagic pancreas (arrow) can be seen. The average mortality from acute pancreatitis is about 10%, with approximately half of the fatalities occurring during the first week of the illness. Patients may die from circulatory collapse, septicaemia, haemorrhage, or respiratory, renal or hepatic failure. Severely ill patients may develop adult respiratory distress syndrome, with tachypnoea, arterial hypoxia and features of shock.

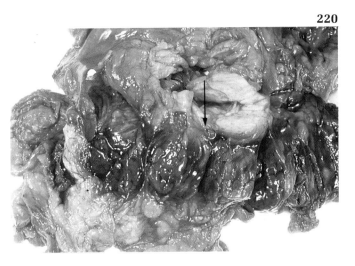

220

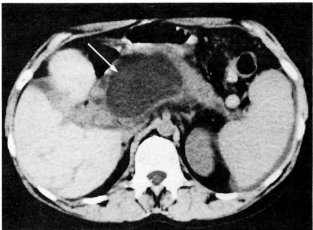

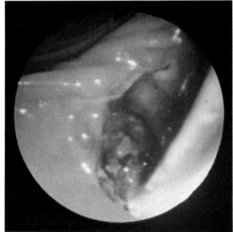

221 Acute pancreatitis. A pseudocyst demonstrated by computerised tomography in a patient with acute pancreatitis (arrow). Pseudocysts are collections of fluid in the pancreas or lesser sac that develop in up to half of the patients who suffer from acute pancreatitis. A pseudocyst should be suspected when an episode of acute pancreatitis fails to settle or recovery is delayed. Pseudocysts may become very large and may give rise to a palpable mass. They usually resolve spontaneously, but they may be complicated by infection or haemorrhage, or may leak into the peritoneal cavity, causing ascites. The treatment of pseudocysts is usually conservative. However, they may require aspiration under ultrasound or computerised tomography guidance. Surgical anastomosis of the pseudocyst to the stomach will relieve the pressure within the pseudocyst and lead to cure.

222 Acute pancreatitis. This view of endoscopic papillotomy and gallstone extraction was obtained from a patient with gallstone pancreatitis. Acute pancreatitis due to gallstones tends to occur in patients who are subsequently found to have multiple small stones which migrate into the common bile duct and may cause oedema of the ampulla, resulting in obstruction of the pancreatic duct. Endoscopic sphincterotomy has the advantage of avoiding major abdominal surgery in an ill patient with pancreatitis. Early reports indicate that this procedure is of value in relieving attacks of acute gallstone pancreatitis, and should certainly be considered in a jaundiced patient with acute pancreatitis.

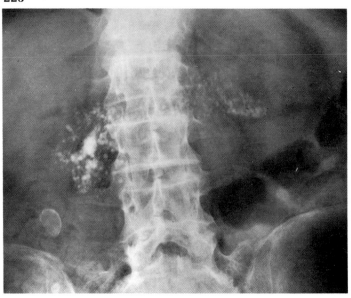

223 Chronic pancreatitis. Calcification throughout the pancreas is seen on this plain upper abdominal radiograph from a patient with alcoholic chronic calcific pancreatitis. Pancreatic calcification is unusual in the common idiopathic form of pancreatitis seen in the West, but may occur in the malnutrition-associated chronic pancreatitis seen in some Asian countries. Occasionally chronic pancreatitis is associated with hyperparathyroidism, hyperlipidaemia or a congenital abnormality of the gland. Chronic pancreatitis usually presents with abdominal or back pain, or both, or may be asymptomatic. Destruction of the exocrine pancreas results in failure of pancreatic enzyme and bicarbonate secretion, leading to maldigestion of fat and steatorrhoea.

224 Chronic pancreatitis. An endoscopic retrograde pancreatogram showing irregularity of the pancreatic duct and mild ectasia of the side-branches (arrow). Not all patients with chronic pancreatitis have an abnormal pancreatogram. The abnormalities are often quite subtle.

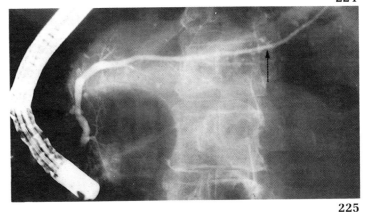

225 Chronic pancreatitis. This endoscopic retrograde pancreatogram demonstrates a dilated main pancreatic duct (arrow).

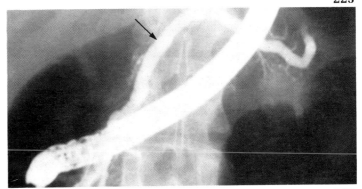

226 Chronic pancreatitis. Computerised tomographic demonstration of the pancreas in a patient with chronic pancreatitis. Note the dilated irregular pancreatic ducts (arrow).

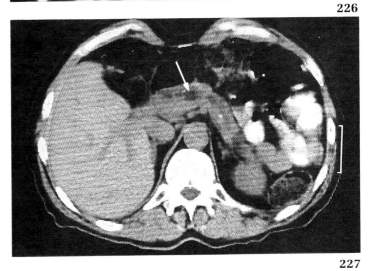

227 Chronic pancreatitis. In this pancreatogram there is mild irregularity of the main pancreatic duct in the head and body of the gland, but the more severe abnormalities are demonstrated in the tail of the gland (upper right) where the main duct and side-branches are markedly dilated. These localised patchy changes are common. The whole pancreas must be filled with contrast during endoscopic pancreatography in order to obtain a correct diagnosis in these patients.

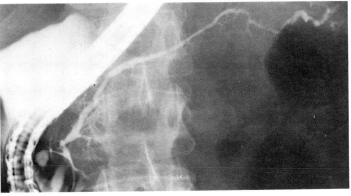

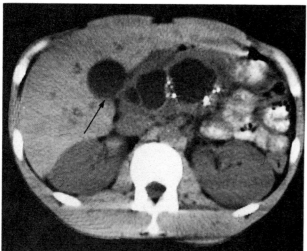

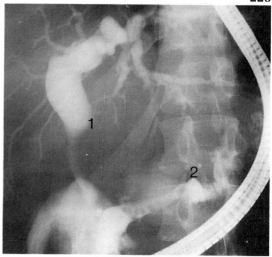

228 Chronic pancreatitis. The changes of gross chronic pancreatitis with calcification and cyst formation are demonstrated in this computerised tomographic scan. Dilated intrahepatic ducts are seen within the liver substance, and the common bile duct is also dilated (arrow) due to obstruction by the diseased pancreas. Cyst formation in chronic pancreatitis may be responsible for an exacerbation of pancreatic pain, and may be relieved by percutaneous aspiration or surgical drainage.

229 Chronic pancreatitis. An endoscopic retrograde cholangiopancreatogram from the same patient as in **228**. The biliary tree is dilated above a smooth stricture (1) caused by compression from the adjacent swollen pancreas. The pancreatic duct is grossly dilated and irregular, and contains multiple radiolucent calculi (2). This alcoholic patient presented with severe abdominal pain and jaundice. He required a Whipple's pancreaticoduodenectomy for relief of these symptoms.

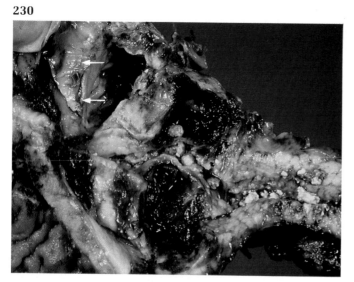

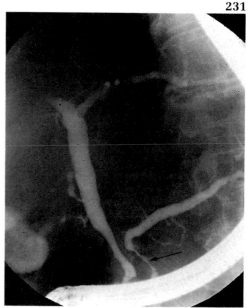

230 Chronic pancreatitis. The resection specimen from the same patient as in **228** and **229**. The pancreas is calcified and the pancreatic duct contains multiple calculi. Cystic areas containing necrotic debris are present in the head of the pancreas. One of these cysts was compressing the common bile duct (arrows). The adjacent duodenum is seen on the bottom left of the photograph.

231 Chronic pancreatitis. This patient was found to have narrowing of the main pancreatic duct in the head of the pancreas at endoscopic retrograde cholangio-pancreatography (arrow). The common bile duct is normal in calibre.

232   Chronic pancreatitis. This 3-day faecal fat collection demonstrates gross steatorrhoea in a patient with exocrine failure due to chronic pancreatitis. Steatorrhoea does not usually develop until approximately 90% of the exocrine pancreas has been destroyed by the chronic inflammatory process. A 3-day faecal fat excretion above 50 g strongly suggests pancreatic insufficiency.

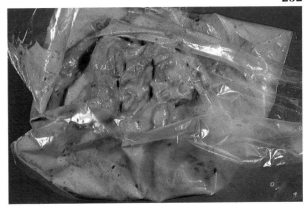

232

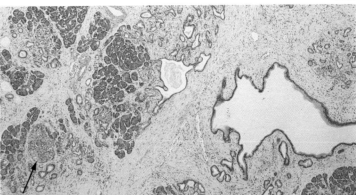

233

233   Chronic pancreatitis. The pancreatic duct is seen on the right of this photomicrograph, and the parenchyma on the left. The lobular duct in the centre is ectatic and contains inspissated eosinophilic, proteinaceous material. The parenchyma is fibrous and there is a relative paucity of exocrine acinar cells, most marked just above the blocked duct in the centre. The exocrine tissue of the pancreas is particularly susceptible to destruction, so the endocrine component appears in relative excess: islets of Langerhans remain prominent at the lower left (arrow).

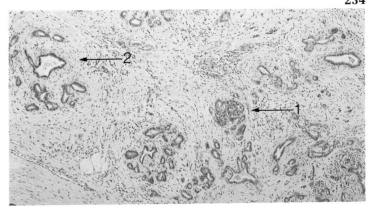

234

234   Chronic pancreatitis. The exocrine tissue in this area of chronic pancreatitis has almost entirely disappeared. All that remains are islands of endocrine tissue (arrow 1), ducts and ductules (arrow 2) trapped within the dense and slightly inflamed fibrous tissue.

235

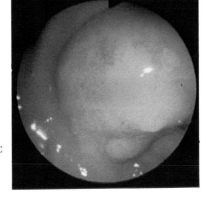

235   Chronic pancreatitis. This view of the second part of the duodenum above the ampulla demonstrates extrinsic compression from a pancreatic cyst. This was found at endoscopic retrograde cholangiopancreatography in a patient with recurrent epigastric pain.

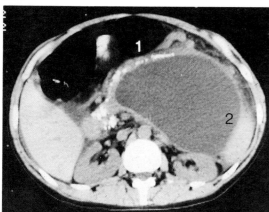
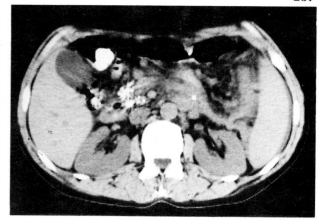

236 and **237** **Chronic pancreatitis.** The computerised tomographic scan in **236** is from a patient with chronic pancreatitis. The calcified gland (1) is displaced by a huge cyst occupying a large portion of the upper abdomen on the left side (2). This cyst was aspirated percutaneously under computerised tomographic control. **237** shows the post-aspiration appearance.

238

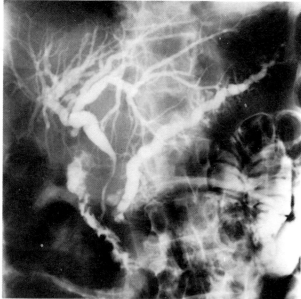

239

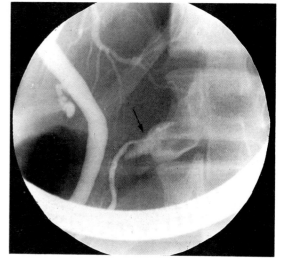

239 **Pancreatic trauma.** An endoscopic retrograde cholangiopancreatogram from a patient involved in a road traffic accident. Contrast stops half-way along the duct, where there is extravasation into the surrounding tissue (arrow). Trauma is usually blunt (for example, due to compression from a car seat belt or steering wheel). Direct penetrating injury by a knife or bullet is rare.

238 **Chronic pancreatitis.** This endoscopic retrograde cholangiopancreatogram was obtained from a patient with chronic pancreatitis and jaundice. The smooth 'rat's tail' stricture of the lower end of the common bile duct is due to chronic pancreatitis. Jaundice may be painless and insidious in patients with alcoholic chronic pancreatitis. Common bile duct compression from chronic pancreatitis may be an unsuspected cause of deterioration in a patient with alcoholic cirrhosis. A serum alkaline phosphatase above three-times normal in a patient with alcoholic cirrhosis suggests a diagnosis of chronic pancreatitis with a low common bile duct stricture. Surgical decompression or endoprosthesis insertion may be necessary to relieve the biliary obstruction.

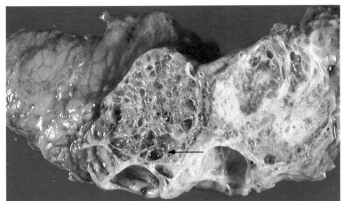

240 Benign pancreatic tumours are less common than malignant tumours. This lesion in the body of pancreas had a variegated and multilocular cut surface and a circumscribed border. There are small as well as larger cysts; some appear haemorrhagic (arrow). Histological examination of this tumour revealed a cystadenoma.

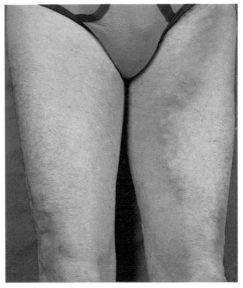

241 Thrombophlebitis. Pancreatic carcinoma usually presents with abdominal pain, progressive jaundice or weight loss. This patient presented with recurrent superficial thrombophlebitis, which may occur in up to 10% of patients with pancreatic carcinoma. Tumours located in the body or tail of the pancreas usually present at an advanced stage with signs of distant spread. Carcinomas of the head of the pancreas classically present with painless progressive jaundice due to common bile duct compression.

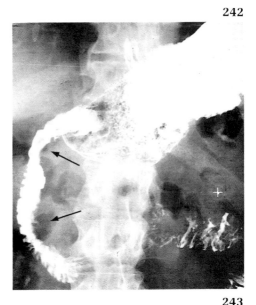

242 Pancreatic carcinoma. A barium meal demonstrating widening of the duodenal loop from extrinsic compression of the second and third parts of the duodenum from a large carcinoma in the head of the pancreas (arrows). This appearance is sometimes referred to as the reverse-3. The tumour may cause nausea, regurgitation or vomiting as a result of duodenal compression. Duodenal obstruction is usually a terminal event, although it may be relieved by performing a gastroenterostomy.

243 Pancreatic carcinoma. A computerised tomographic scan showing advanced carcinoma of the head of the pancreas (1) with hepatic metastases (2). The large pancreatic mass is seen anteriorly. There are two large hepatic metastases in the right lobe of the liver. The anterior metastases contain a rim of calcification. Calcified hepatic metastases are unusual in pancreatic carcinoma and are more commonly seen in patients with carcinoma of the colon. Computerised tomographic scanning and ultrasound have improved diagnostic precision in patients with carcinoma of the pancreas, but have failed to make any impact on the dismal outlook for patients with this disease, because the tumour is usually advanced when symptoms develop.

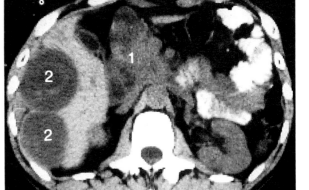

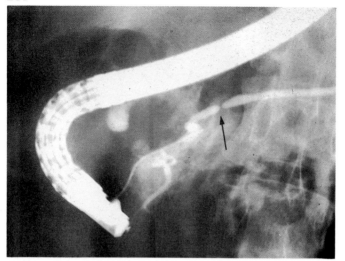

244 Pancreatic carcinoma. This endoscopic retrograde pancreatogram has opacified the main pancreatic duct and demonstrated a small stricture compressing the duct (arrow). The differential diagnosis for a stricture of this kind includes pancreatic carcinoma and chronic pancreatitis. This appearance has also been described as a normal variant. Endoscopic retrograde cholangiopancreatography is valuable in patients with suspected pancreatic carcinoma, especially if ultrasound suggests obstructive jaundice. Samples of pancreatic juice may be obtained for cytological examination.

245

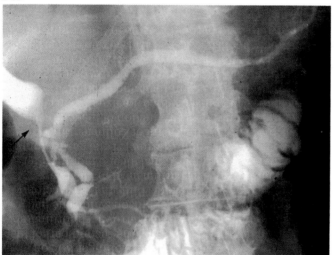

245 Pancreatic carcinoma. This endoscopic retrograde cholangiopancreatogram is characteristic of a carcinoma in the head of the pancreas. There is a stricture of the pancreatic duct, which also involves the common bile duct. The common bile duct is dilated above the stricture (arrow).

246

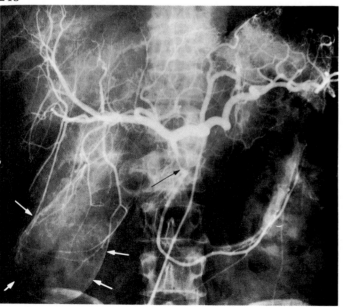

246 Pancreatic carcinoma. Arteriography can be useful in assessing the extent of tumour mass in patients for whom surgical resection is being considered, and it occasionally identifies tumours where other techniques have failed. This study has demonstrated a carcinoma of the head of the pancreas, which is compressing the superior mesenteric artery (arrow). The patient also had obstructive jaundice with a palpable gall bladder. The position of the distended gall bladder has been shown on this radiograph (arrows).

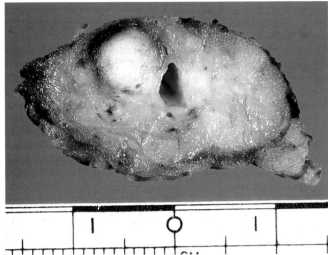

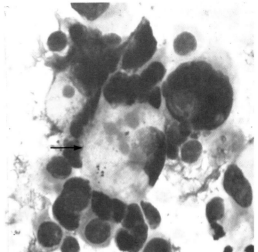

247 Pancreatic carcinoma. A small tumour above and to the left of the splenic vein (centre) in the body of the pancreas. Although the tumour appears rounded, its edges are ill-defined and there is haemorrhage around its upper border. The pancreas has lost its lobular architecture and is paler than usual. The tumour was seen microscopically to be a poorly differentiated adenocarcinoma. Much of the pallor of the tumour and adjacent pancreas is attributable to the dense fibrosis that often accompanies these carcinomas.

248 Pancreatic carcinoma. Fine-needle aspiration cytology of a pancreatic adenocarcinoma stained by the MGG technique. The large tumour cell is distended by its content of mucus (arrow). This clump of cells shows the typical cytological features of malignancy: hyperchromatism, pleomorphism and nuclear chromatin clumping.

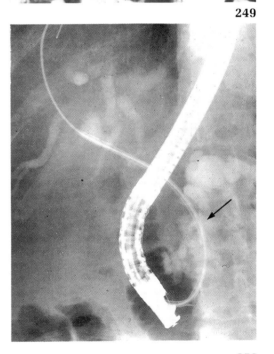

249 Pancreatic carcinoma. The treatment of pancreatic carcinoma is unsatisfactory. An attempt at curative resection should only be considered in patients who are sufficiently fit to tolerate the procedure and whose tumour appears to be less than 3 cm in size without obvious metastases. Palliation of the symptoms of obstructive jaundice may be achieved surgically or by means of a biliary endoprosthesis. This may be inserted percutaneously or endoscopically. The figure shows the endoscopic passage of an endoprosthesis (arrow) over a guide wire through the ampulla of Vater and into the biliary system. The guide wire is then withdrawn and the prosthesis is left in place.

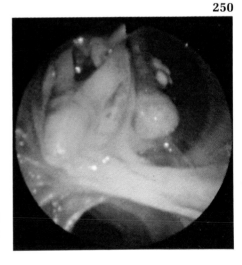

250 Pancreatic carcinoma. This endoscopic view demonstrates invasion of the third part of the duodenum by a large carcinoma of the pancreas (arrow). The tip of the endoprosthesis may be seen emerging from the ampulla of Vater. Biliary endoprostheses have a tendency to block, and may require removal and substitution approximately every 6 months. The endoprosthesis was blocked in this patient, but was successfully changed endoscopically.

251

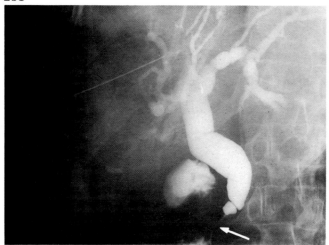

251 Pancreatic carcinoma. Percutaneous transhepatic cholangiography has shown dilatation of the biliary system and a tight stricture at the lower end of the common bile duct, due to a carcinoma of the head of the pancreas (arrow).

252

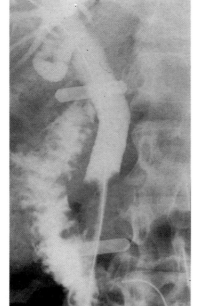

253

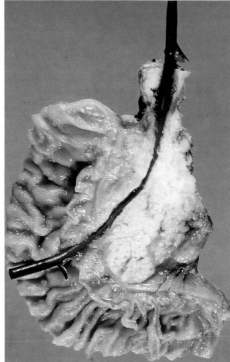

252 Pancreatic carcinoma. A guide wire has been inserted percutaneously, through the dilated intrahepatic bile duct and the malignant stricture at the lower end of the common bile duct into the duodenum. This internal–external biliary drain was later substituted by an endoprosthesis.

253 Pancreatic carcinoma. This post-mortem photograph demonstrates the position of a biliary endoprosthesis in a patient who died from a carcinoma of the head of the pancreas but remained free of jaundice. The small projections on the endoprosthesis prevent displacement.

254

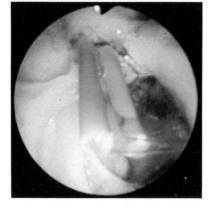

254 Pancreatic carcinoma. An endoscopic view of the ampulla, showing free drainage of bile from two endoprostheses that have been inserted into the biliary system to bypass a malignant obstruction.

255 Pancreatic carcinoma.
A photomicrograph of moderately
differentiated adenocarcinoma of
the head of pancreas set within
dense fibrous tissue.

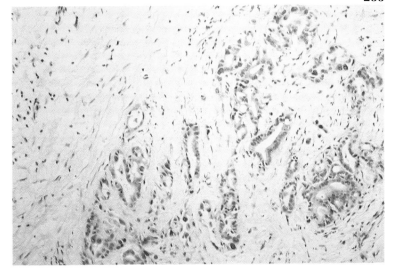

256 Pancreatic carcinoma. The
same tumour as **255**, stained by an
immunoperoxidase method for
carcino-embryonic antigen. The
expression of this marker by these
tumour cells and its measurement
in the serum is sometimes of
value in the diagnosis and follow-
up of patients with pancreatic
carcinoma.

257 Pancreatic carcinoma. The
same tumour as in **255** and **256**,
stained with an
immunoperoxidase technique
using RE20. This polyclonal
antibody is directed against a
mixture of low molecular weight
cytokeratins; these may assist in
the histological identification of
pancreatic carcinomas.

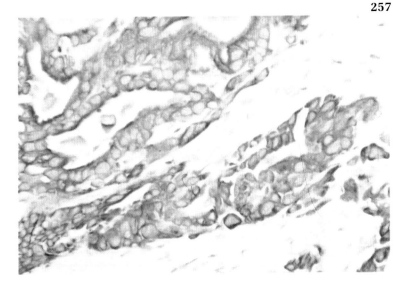

258

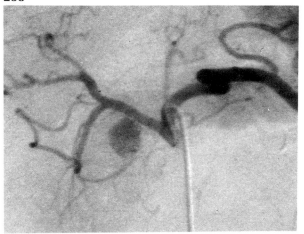

258 Hormone-secreting pancreatic tumours. These arise from the APUD cells, a group of endocrine cells within the pancreas. These tumours may be benign or malignant, and may give rise to many clinical syndromes resulting from the inappropriate secretion of different peptide hormones. Insulinomas arise from the beta-cells of the pancreatic islets. They present with hypoglycyaemia that develops during fasting or after exercise. Arteriography may detect up to 90% of insulinomas. This coeliac axis digital subtraction arteriogram has demonstrated a rounded tumour in the head of the pancreas. Surgical excision resulted in complete cure.

259

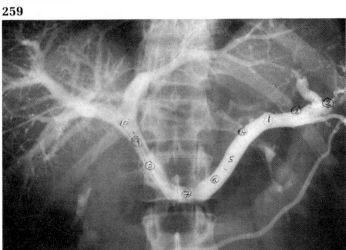

260

259 and 260 Hormone-secreting pancreatic tumours. The localisation of small hormone-secreting pancreatic tumours may prove difficult. These figures illustrate the technique of percutaneous transhepatic portal venous sampling. Contrast has been injected into the hepatic and splenic venous systems (**259**) and into the superior mesenteric vein (**260**). Separate samples of venous blood have been obtained from each of the sites numbered on the radiograph. The site from which the maximum hormone concentration is obtained may indicate the part of the pancreas containing the tumour. Selective venous sampling is very helpful for localising insulinomas and glucagonomas, but has been less successful for identifying gastrinomas.

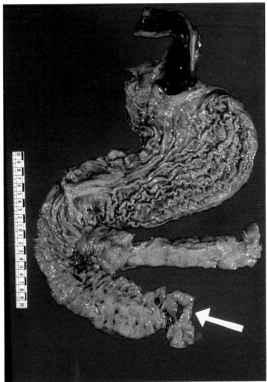

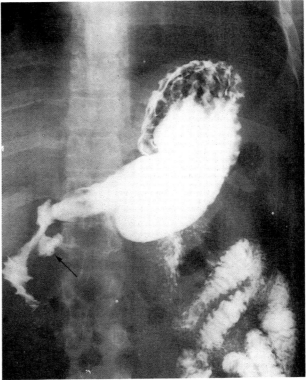

261 Zollinger Ellison syndrome. This syndrome arises from the commonest hormone-secreting tumour of the pancreas, the gastrinoma. Secretion of gastrin may lead to intractable peptic ulceration from gastric acid hypersecretion. Gastrinomas may be part of the familial multiple endocrine neoplasia type I syndrome in about 25% of patients. In this post-mortem photograph a gastrinoma is seen in the head of the pancreas, and there are multiple perforations of the third part of the duodenum (arrow) as a result of gastric acid hypersecretion.

A basal gastric acid output of more than 20 mmol/h is highly suggestive of a gastrinoma. Fasting hypergastrinaemia is almost always present and rises with the administration of intravenous secretin. Localisation of gastrinomas is notoriously difficult, but attempts should be made to localise the tumour with ultrasonography, computerised tomographic scanning, arteriography and percutaneous transhepatic selective venous sampling. Laparotomy will only detect the tumour in about 70% of patients. Liver metastases are common.

262 and 263   Zollinger Ellison syndrome. 262 is a barium meal in a patient with Zollinger Ellison syndrome. An ulcer crater in the second part of the duodenum is demonstrated (arrow). Unfortunately the diagnosis of Zollinger Ellison syndrome had not been considered, and a Billroth II gastrectomy was performed. The barium meal in **263** has demonstrated a large stomal ulcer 6 months after the partial gastrectomy (arrow). Total gastrectomy was the standard treatment of Zollinger Ellison syndrome until the introduction of histamine H_2-receptor antagonists, which are usually successful in controlling the symptoms and complications of gastric acid hypersecretion. Recently omeprazole, a hydrogen–potassium-ATPase inhibitor that virtually abolishes gastric acid secretion, has been shown to be of particular value in this condition.

263

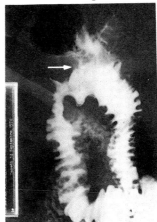
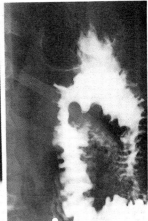

264

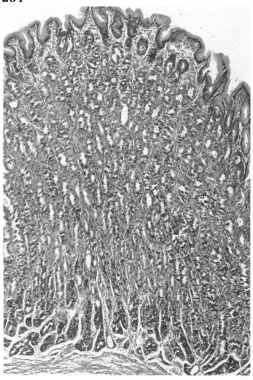

265

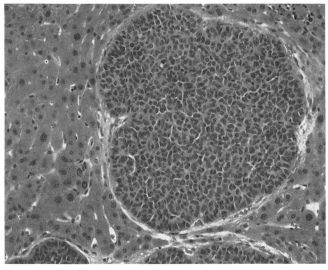

265 Zollinger Ellison syndrome. These rounded islands of cells are liver metastases from an endocrine tumour originating in the pancreas.

264 Zollinger Ellison syndrome. Gastric body mucosa from a patient with Zollinger Ellison syndrome. The specialised glands of the gastric body show marked hyperplasia, and oxyphilic cells are increased. In this case (also seen in **265** and **266**) the stimulation of the acid-secreting epithelium was a direct consequence of gastrin secretion from a pancreatic endocrine tumour.

266

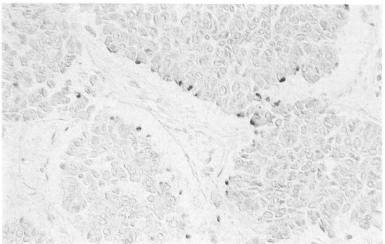

266 Zollinger Ellison syndrome. The same tumour as **265**, stained by an immunoperoxidase technique for gastrin. The brown-stained cells contain the hormone.

CHAPTER 7

The Normal Small Intestine

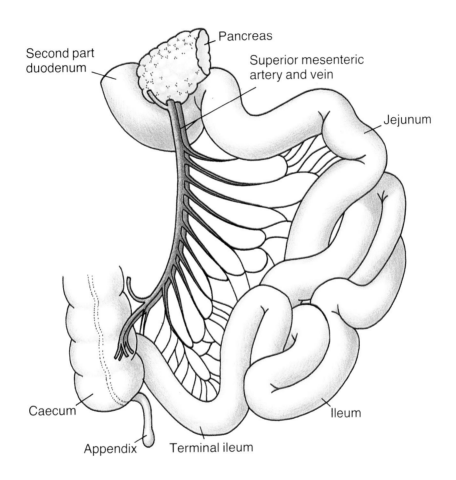

The normal small intestine includes the duodenum, jejunum and ileum. The whole small intestine is approximately 6 m long. The mesentery from which the jejunum and ileum are suspended contain branches of the superior mesenteric artery and vein, as well as numerous autonomic nerve fibres and lymphatics. The length of the small intestine and the presence of the transverse valvuli conniventes serve to increase the epithelial surface area, enabling maximum absorption of nutrients and water from its lumen. Absorption of amino acids, oligopeptides, monosaccharides, fatty acids, iron, folic acid, and other vitamins and minerals, occurs mainly in the jejunum. The terminal ileum is responsible for absorption of vitamin B_{12} and reabsorption of bile salts.

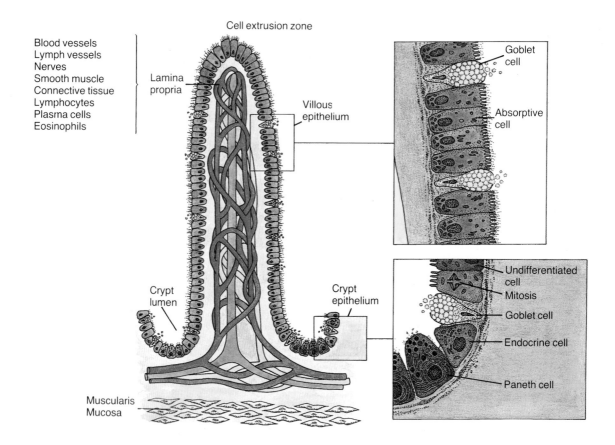

Cell extrusion zone

Blood vessels
Lymph vessels
Nerves
Smooth muscle
Connective tissue
Lymphocytes
Plasma cells
Eosinophils

Lamina propria

Villous epithelium

Goblet cell

Absorptive cell

Crypt lumen

Crypt epithelium

Undifferentiated cell

Mitosis

Goblet cell

Endocrine cell

Paneth cell

Muscularis Mucosa

Schematic diagrams showing the histological organisation of the mucosa of the small intestine at different magnifications. Characteristics of normal jejunal tissue are: long villi, shallow crypts and appropriate cellularity in the lamina propria (compare with **274** and **277**).

267 Normal small intestine. The jejunum and ileum are essential for normal life because of their digestive and absorptive functions. Their structure is assessed by means of a small bowel meal. Barium is swallowed by the patient and screened during its passage through the loops of the jejunum and ileum. The transit time through the small intestine varies greatly between normal individuals. The circular valvuli conniventes are clearly seen. The right colon has started to fill.

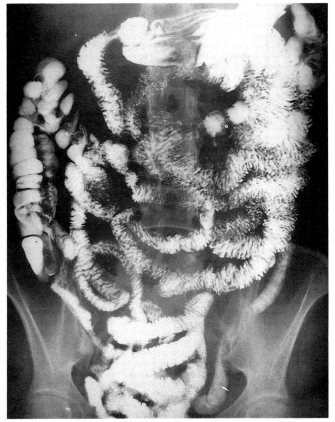

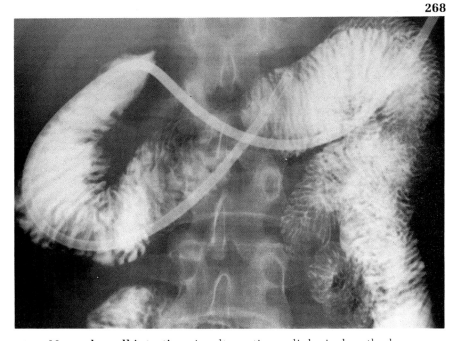

268 Normal small intestine. An alternative radiological method of imaging the small intestine is the small bowel enema (small bowel enteroclysis). A nasogastric tube is guided into the fourth part of the duodenum, allowing infusion of barium suspension directly into the jejunum. This double-contrast technique is useful for identifying strictures or fine mucosal lesions.

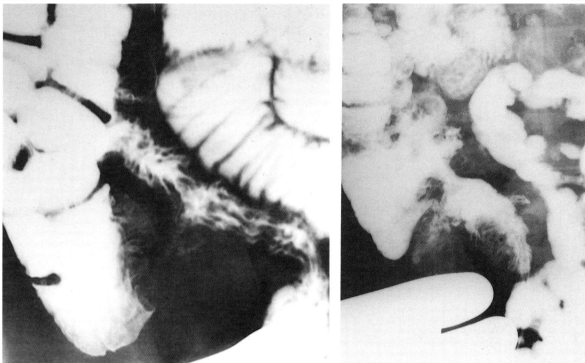

269A and B   Normal terminal ileum. This small bowel meal has demonstrated a normal terminal ileum and caecum. The normal feathery mucosal pattern of the terminal ileum is seen. Overlying small bowel loops may impede the visualisation of the terminal ileum, and the radiologist may need to apply external manipulation to enable clear views to be obtained (**269B**). Air-contrast views of the terminal ileal mucosa can be obtained by insufflation of air through a rectal catheter during this procedure.

270

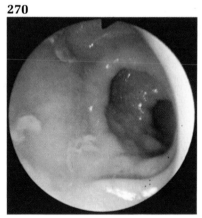

270   Normal terminal ileum, as shown after passage of a colonoscope through the ileo-caecal valve.

271 to **273**   **Jejunal biopsy.** The Crosby capsule is used to obtain a biopsy sample. The capsule is a small metal cylinder with a 3 mm port attached to a length of hollow tubing. It is swallowed by the patient and guided into the jejunum. The position of the capsule is checked by screening (**273**). Once in position, abrupt aspiration is applied to the hollow tubing, and a small portion of mucosa is sucked through the port into the capsule. A spring-loaded rotating knife within the cylinder slices off the biopsy sample and the apparatus is withdrawn.

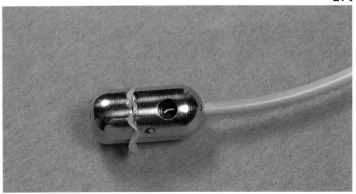

271

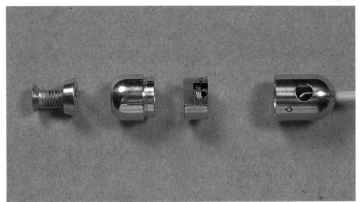

272

273

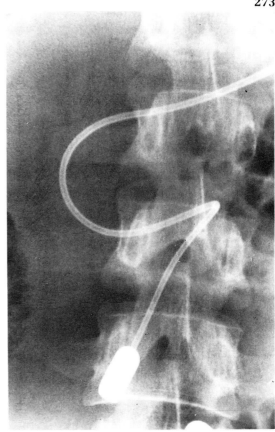

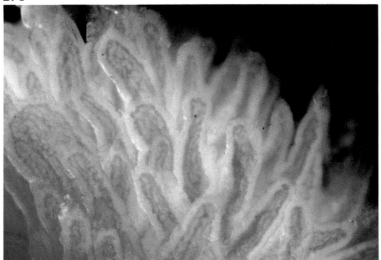

274　Normal jejunal biopsy. This dissecting micrograph of jejunal mucosa shows the normal villous pattern. As will be seen in Chapter 8, this morphology is readily distinguishable from the villous atrophy seen in coeliac disease (**283**).

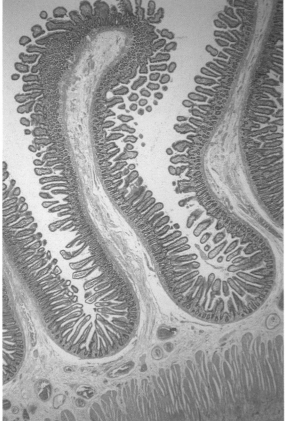

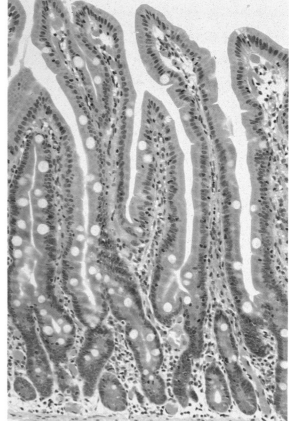

275　Normal jejunal biopsy. This is a longitudinal section to show the small intestinal folds covered by normal mucosa. The transverse circular folds and the mucosal villi both contribute towards increasing the absorptive epithelial surface area of the jejunum.

276　Normal jejunal mucosa. Long, slender villi are seen. These are usually slightly shorter than the villi of the duodenum.

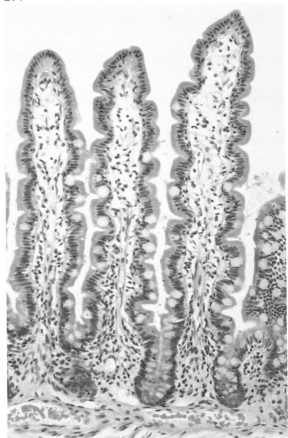

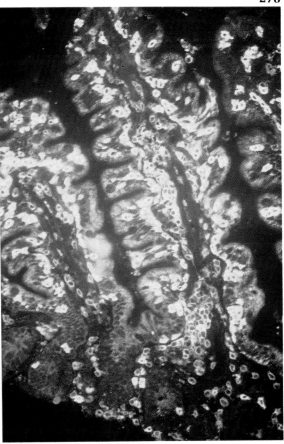

277 Normal ileal mucosa. Ileal villi are generally a little shorter and broader than in the more proximal parts of the small intestine.

278 Normal jejunum. This is a double-label immunofluorescence preparation using monoclonal antibodies to CD3 ('pan-T', green) and CD8 (cytotoxic/suppressor subset). The cells labelled green are of the helper/inducer T-lymphocyte subset. The cells labelled yellow are of the cytotoxic/suppressor T-lymphocyte subset. The majority of T-cells in the intra-epithelial compartment are of the suppressor/cytotoxic (CD8) subset. This contrasts with the lamina propria subset distribution, where the helper/inducer T-lymphocyte subset predominates.

CHAPTER 8

Diseases of the Small Intestine

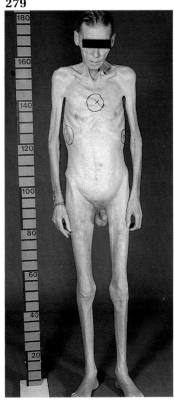

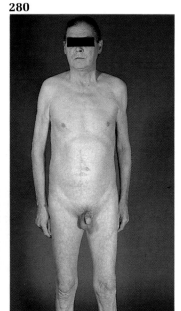

279 and **280   Coeliac disease.** This disease is the most common and most important cause of malabsorption in the West. It is characterised by partial or subtotal jejunal villous atrophy which improves morphologically when treated with a gluten-free diet, and which deteriorates again on reintroduction of gluten. This patient presented with combined iron and folic acid deficiency and severe emaciation. After 4 months' treatment with a gluten-free diet he had gained 23 kg in weight and his anaemia had resolved.

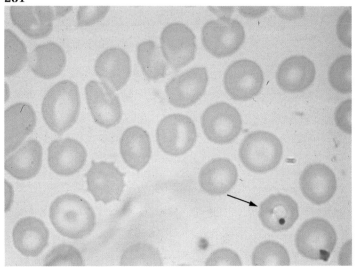

281   Coeliac disease. The diagnosis may be suggested by the appearance of the peripheral blood film. Combined iron and folic acid deficiencies give rise to a dimorphic picture in which macrocytic and microcytic red cells coexist. Furthermore, splenic atrophy occurs in about one-third of patients with coeliac disease, leading to the appearance of target cells and Howell–Jolly bodies (small, dense, basophilic nuclear remnants within red cells; arrow). This blood film from a patient with coeliac disease shows all of these features.

282 Coeliac disease. The small bowel meal x-ray is usually abnormal in coeliac disease. The mucosa becomes featureless and tubular, and the normal fine feathery appearance of the mucosa is lost (compare with **268**). There may be flocculation of barium. These small bowel meal appearances are entirely non-specific, but they may suggest or confirm a clinical suspicion of malabsorption.

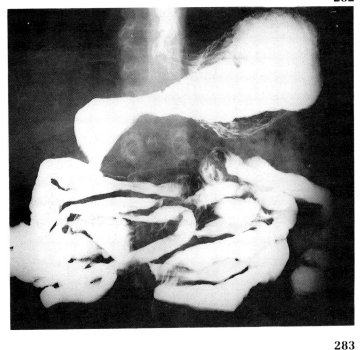

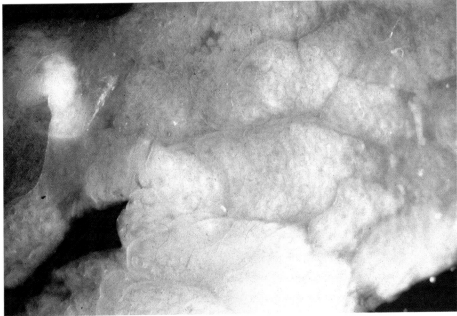

283 Coeliac disease. The dissecting microscopic appearance of the jejunal mucosa in untreated coeliac disease shows a loss of the normal villous architecture and subtotal villous atrophy. Compare this mosaic appearance with the normal jejunal mucosa (**274**).

284

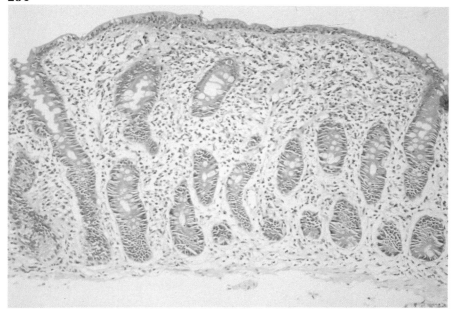

285

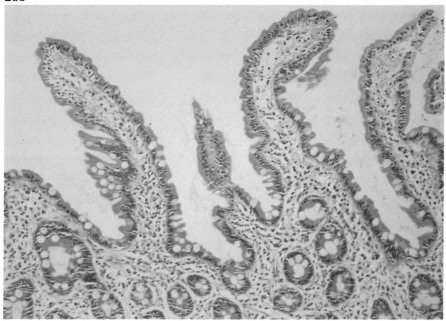

284 and **285** **Coeliac disease.** Jejunal biopsy of a patient with untreated coeliac disease (**284**). There is an increase in mononuclear inflammatory cells in the lamina propria and an increase in intra-epithelial small lymphocytes. The villi have almost entirely disappeared. Following gluten withdrawal (**285**) there is a decrease in lamina proprial inflammatory cells and intra-epithelial lymphocytes, and villi have reformed.

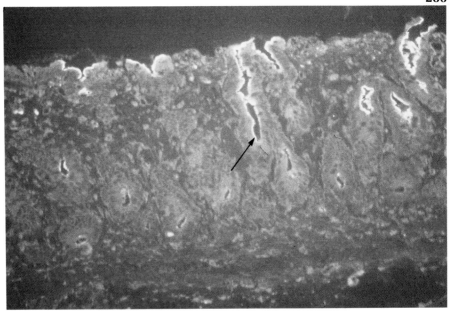

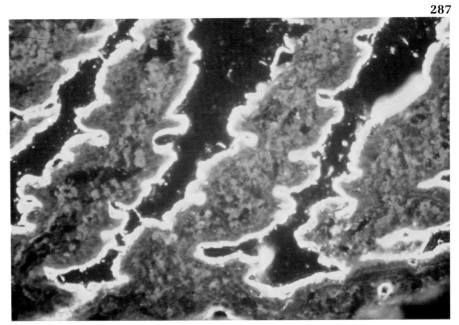

286 and **287   Coeliac disease.** The common acute lymphoblastic
leukaemia antigen (CALLA) is a marker of the brush-border of jejunal
enterocytes (yellow fluorescence on epithelial surface). **286** is a jejunal
biopsy from a patient with untreated coeliac disease. There are no villi,
and the damaged surface enterocytes have virtually lost all expression of
CALLA, which is only detectable in crypt epithelium (arrow). **287** is a
jejunal biopsy following gluten withdrawal and return to normal
histological appearances. The CALLA expression pattern had also
returned to normal, indicating repair of brush-border damage.

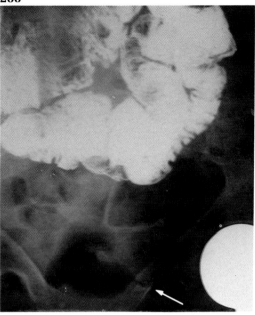

288 Coeliac disease. A small bowel meal has been performed in the investigation of an elderly woman with malabsorption. There is a pseudofracture of the superior pubic ramus on the left side (arrow). This skeletal abnormality is termed a Looser's zone and is typical of osteomalacia resulting from vitamin D and calcium malabsorption. Bone pain and limb girdle weakness may be presenting features of coeliac disease with osteomalacia.

289

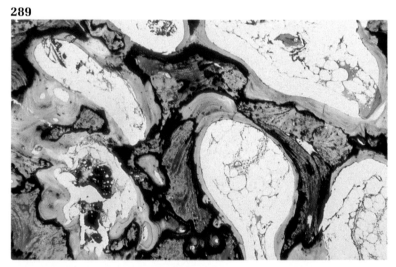

289 Osteomalacia. A bone biopsy from the iliac crest prepared by the Tripp and McKay technique. The border of the calcified bone trabeculae and unmineralised osteoid are outlined in black. Many of the bony trabeculae have a thick covering of osteoid. This appearance is characteristic of osteomalacia.

290

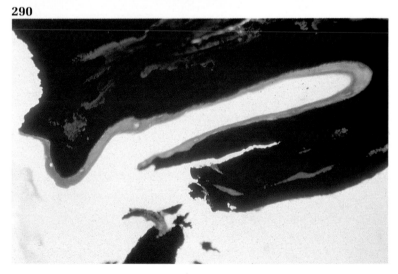

290 Osteomalacia. The same case of osteomalacia as in **289**, seen at higher magnification. Calcified bone (black) is covered by a thick coat of osteoid.

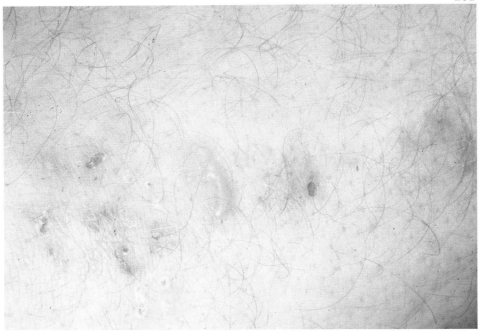

291 Dermatitis herpetiformis. This skin eruption is characterised by intensely itchy papular or vesicular lesions that lie on an urticarial or erythematous base. The elbows, knees, sacrum and shoulders are the most commonly affected sites. About 20% of patients with dermatitis herpetiformis have coeliac disease. The presence of both disorders in the same patient is linked genetically with the presence of human leucocyte antigens B8 and DR3. Sometimes patients with dermatitis herpetiformis have no symptoms to suggest coeliac disease, but are found to have mild or moderate jejunal mucosal abnormalities. Treatment with a gluten-free diet may ameliorate the skin condition.

292 Dermatitis herpetiformis. This patient with coeliac disease had an itchy maculopapular eruption of the sacral skin. Although dermatitis herpetiformis is classified as a bullous disorder, the blisters are usually not seen, as they are scratched by the patient in an effort to relieve the pruritus. The dermatitis responds to a combination of a gluten-free diet and oral dapsone treatment.

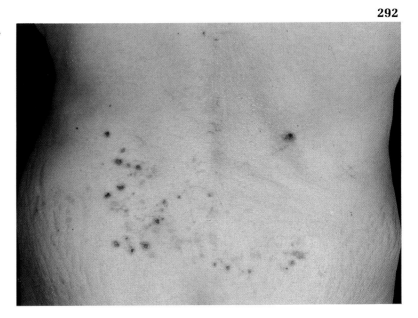

293

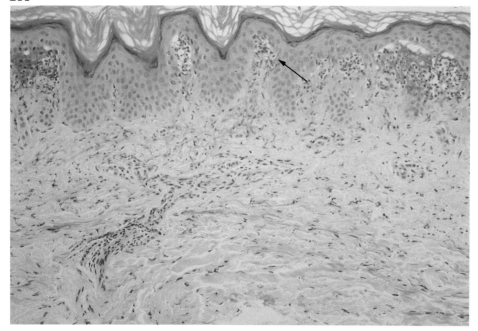

293 Dermatitis herpetiformis. Photomicrograph of a section of skin from a patient with dermatitis herpetiformis in association with coeliac disease. This is an early lesion with four separate micro-abscesses located at the tips of the dermal papillae (arrow). In later lesions the micro-abscesses coalesce so that a bulla is formed with a plane of separation at the dermo-epidermal junction.

294

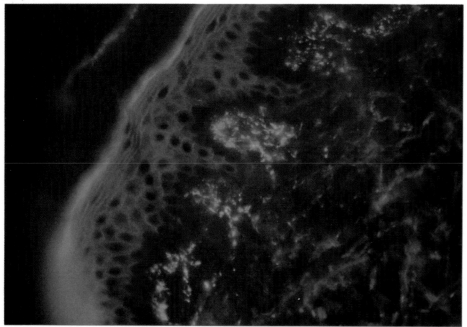

294 Dermatitis herpetiformis. An immunofluorescent technique has identified granular deposits of IgA at the dermo-epidermal junction and in the dermal papillae. These deposits are characteristic of dermatitis herpetiformis.

295 Intestinal lymphangiectasia. An operative photograph of loops of small bowel with prominent pale lymphatics apparent on the serosal surface in a patient with intestinal lymphangiectasia. This disorder may be primary, or secondary to blockage of the lymphatic drainage of the small bowel (for example, malignant disease). A protein-losing enteropathy with leg oedema and hypoalbuminaemia is the usual clinical presentation. Ascites or pleural effusions may occur. The diagnosis is normally made by jejunal biopsy. Treatment involves the reduction of lymphatic flow by restricting dietary long-chain triglycerides and replacing them with medium-chain triglycerides.

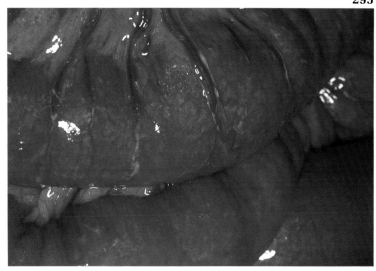

296

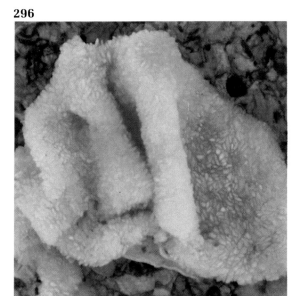

297

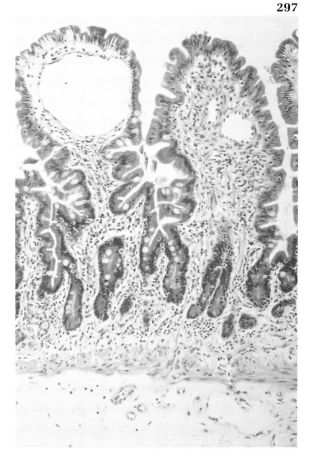

296 Intestinal lymphangiectasia. A full-thickness biopsy of the small bowel from the same patient as **295**, viewed from the mucosal surface, shows distension and clubbing of the villi due to the ectatic (fat-filled) lacteals within them.

297 Intestinal lymphangiectasia. Dilated superficial lymphatics within the villi of the small bowel are seen in this histological section.

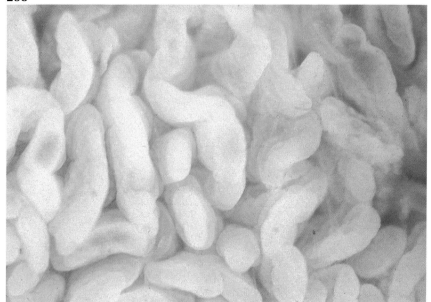

298 Tropical sprue. This form of post-infective malabsorption usually occurs in patients who are living in or have recently returned from the Indian subcontinent, South-East Asia, Central America or parts of Africa. The disorder occasionally develops in people who have always lived in subtropical or even temperate climates. The usual presenting complaint is persistent diarrhoea after an acute gastrointestinal infection. The patient loses weight and the stools become bulky, pale and fatty. Partial villous atrophy of the jejunal mucosa develops. The figure is a dissecting micrograph of a jejunal biopsy in a patient with tropical sprue. There is partial villous atrophy, and villous fusion resulting in broad "leaf-like" forms.

299

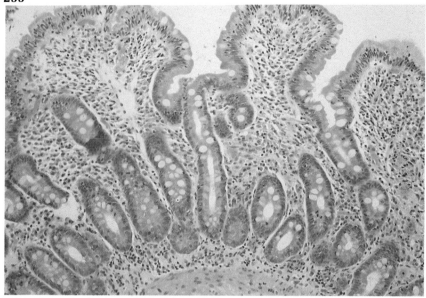

299 Tropical sprue. This jejunal biopsy section displays an increase in chronic inflammatory cells in the lamina propria and an excess of small lymphocytes within the epithelium. The villi are short and broad. These are the features of partial villous atrophy (crypt hyperplastic type). Tetracycline and folic acid are valuable in the treatment of tropical sprue.

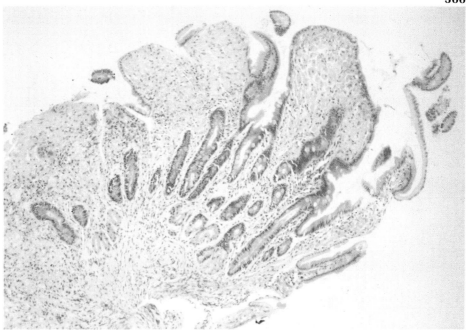

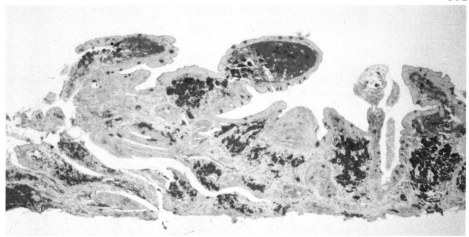

300 and **301**   **Whipple's disease.** This very rare disease is associated with the presence of Gram-negative bacilli within foamy macrophages in the lamina propria of the small intestine. Malabsorption is the usual presenting feature. The lamina propria in the jejunal biopsy in **300** is expanded and the villi have become club-shaped due to the presence of large numbers of foamy macrophages. These have been stained with the PAS technique in **301**, and show an intense red colour.

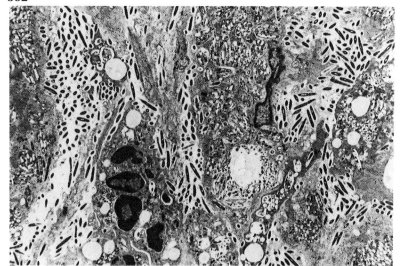

302

302 and 303 Whipple's disease. 302 Electron microscopic examination of lamina propria macrophages has revealed numerous rod-shaped bacteria. The structure of Whipple's bacilli is seen in more detail at higher power in **303**.

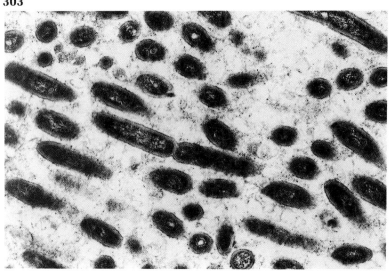

303

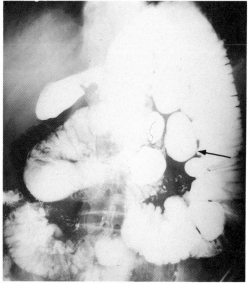

304

304 Small bowel diverticulosis. This barium meal and follow-through demonstrates multiple large jejunal diverticula (arrow). These are herniations of jejunal mucosa through the muscle coat of the bowel wall, and are usually asymptomatic. Sometimes stagnation occurs with proliferation of bacteria within the diverticula, and this may lead to malabsorption of vitamin B_{12} and deconjugation of bile salts. It is sometimes difficult to be certain whether jejunal diverticulosis is directly responsible for malabsorption in individual patients. A ^{14}C glycocholate acid breath test or direct aspiration of the jejunum for bacteriology may assist the investigation of patients with malabsorption and jejunal diverticula. Small intestinal bacterial overgrowth may also follow the formation of surgical blind loops. Broad-spectrum antibiotics, such as tetracycline, are used for the treatment of small intestinal bacterial overgrowth, but repeated courses or life-long therapy may be necessary.

305 Jejunal diverticulosis.
A post-mortem photograph
showing extensive jejunal
diverticulosis. Diverticula of
the small intestine are usually
wide-mouthed.

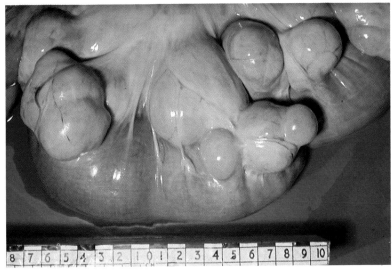

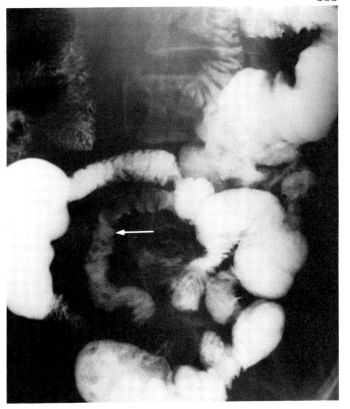

306 Amyloidosis. This disease results
from the extracellular deposition of
amyloid protein throughout the body.
Amyloidosis may be primary or may
occur in association with diseases such
as multiple myeloma, osteomyelitis or
familial Mediterranean fever. The
amyloid fibrils may be deposited widely
in the gastrointestinal tract, leading to
diarrhoea, malabsorption or protein-
losing enteropathy. This barium follow-
through examination in a patient with
small intestinal amyloidosis showed
sluggish transit of barium through the
intestine, with thickened nodular folds
in one loop (arrow). The diagnosis of
amyloidosis depends on histological
examination of the involved tissue.
Rectal biopsy will provide the diagnosis
in about 80% of patients with diffuse
disease. Peroral endoscopic biopsy of
stomach or small intestine may provide
positive results in some cases with a
negative rectal biopsy.

307

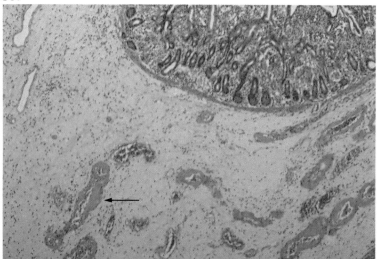

307 Amyloidosis. The mucosa and submucosa of a patient with widespread amyloidosis in association with myeloma. Staining with haematoxylin and eosin reveals a homogeneous dark pink thickening of the walls of the submucosal blood vessels (arrow).

308

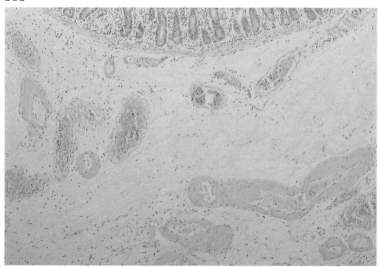

308 Amyloidosis. Another section from the same patient as **307**, stained with Congo Red. The abnormal material in the walls of the submucosal blood vessels appears light orange.

309

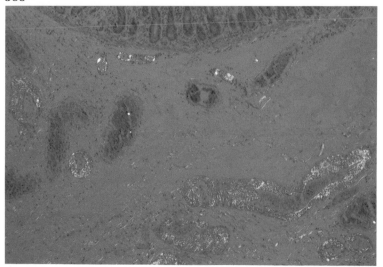

309 Amyloidosis. The same field as **308** in polarised light. Abnormal congophilic material can now be seen to show a green–yellow birefringence. Amyloid deposits characteristically have an affinity for Congo Red dye and show 'apple-green' birefringence when viewed in polarised light.

310 to **312**　**Amyloidosis.** A rectal biopsy from the same patient as **307** to **309**. The eosinophilic deposits of amyloid around blood vessels in the superficial lamina propria is only just visible with conventional staining. Nevertheless, this material shows affinity for Congo Red and characteristic apple-green birefringence when viewed in polarised light.

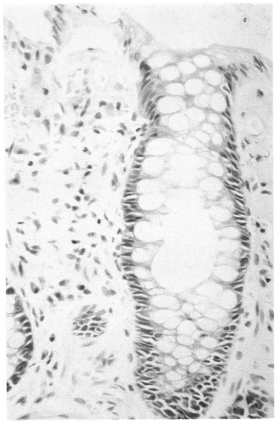

311

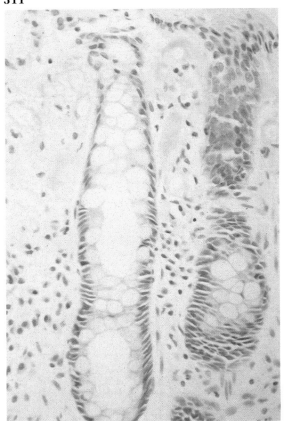

312

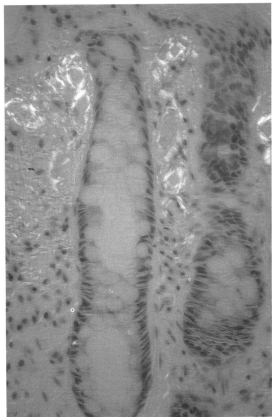

313

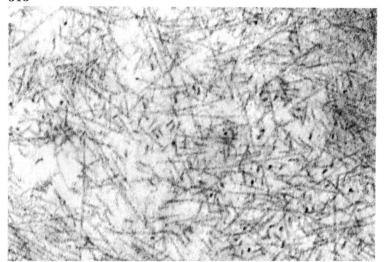

313 Amyloidosis. This electron micrograph demonstrates the morphology of amyloid fibrils. The infiltrate is composed of linear, haphazardly arranged, non-branching fibrils averaging 10 nm in diameter (orig. mag. ×46,000).

314

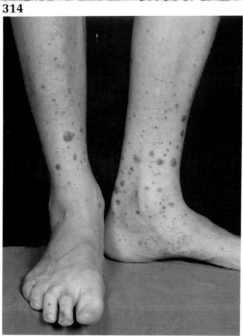

314 and 315 Henoch–Schonlein purpura. This is typically a disease of prepubertal boys, with the majority aged 6 months to 6 years, although it can occur in adults. It is characterised by the tetrad of a purpuric rash, colicky abdominal pain (with or without bloody diarrhoea), arthralgia and glomerulonephritis. The organ involvement may develop in any chronological order. The vasculitic rash tends to involve the feet, the extensor surfaces of the legs, and the buttocks. The disease is often self-limiting, but complications such as rapidly progressive renal failure or gastrointestinal haemorrhage may warrant therapeutic intervention.

315

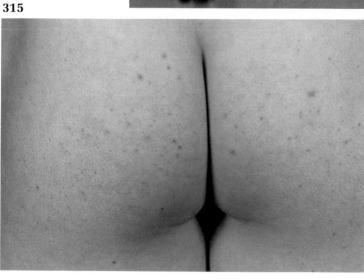

316   **317**

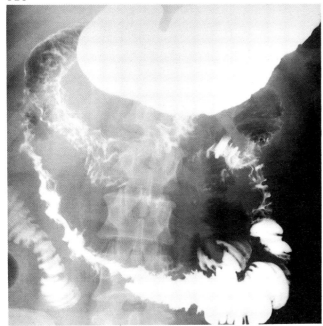

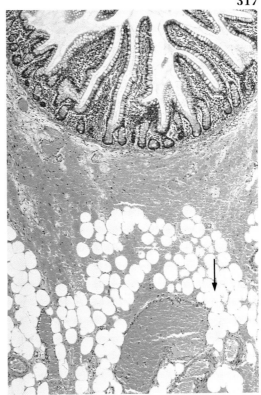

316   **Henoch–Schonlein purpura.** A barium follow-through x-ray showing narrowing and ulceration of several loops of small intestine in a patient with gastrointestinal bleeding. The jejunum and ileum are most commonly involved. This unusual appearance mimics Crohn's disease or lymphoma.

318

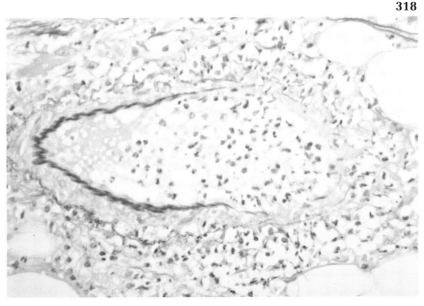

317 and **318**   **Henoch–Schonlein purpura.** Photomicrographs of a resected segment of small bowel from a patient with gastrointestinal bleeding. There is extensive recent haemorrhage into the submucosa. A cluster of small submucosal blood vessels is seen in the lower right of **317** (arrow). **318** is a high-power view of one of these blood vessels. The preparation has been stained to demonstrate elastin in black and collagen in red. There has been acute inflammatory destruction of the vessel wall on the right of the field, as demonstrated by the disintegration of the elastic layer. This vasculitic process underlies the haemorrhagic manifestations of Henoch–Schonlein purpura.

111

319

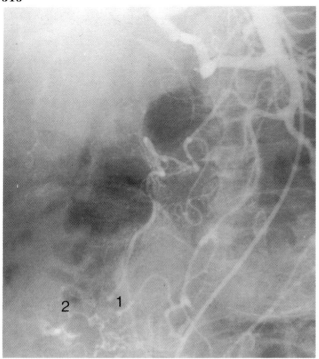

319 Polyarteritis nodosa. Polyarteritis is an inflammatory disorder of medium- and small- sized arteries. Nausea, vomiting, abdominal pain, weight loss and diarrhoea are common symptoms. Occasionally gastrointestinal bleeding or focal intestinal infarction may occur. This superior mesenteric arteriogram was performed in a patient with gastrointestinal bleeding. There are micro-aneurysms of the medium-sized arteries (1) and a bleeding point is seen in the right iliac fossa (2).

320   **321**

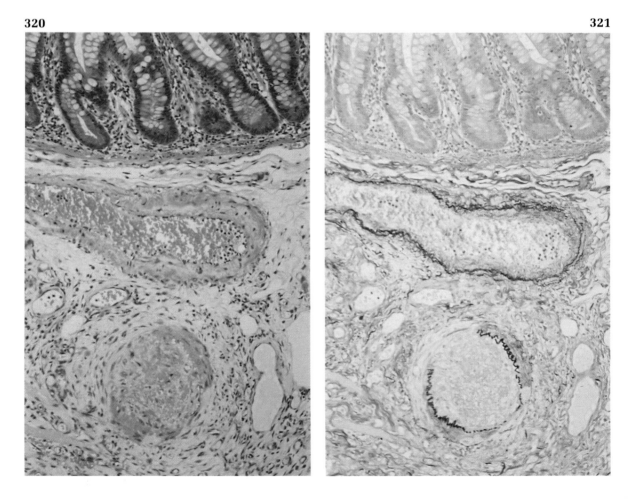

320 to **322** **Polyarteritis nodosa.**
Photomicrographs of the mucosa and submucosa
of the small bowel of a patient with polyarteritis
nodosa. The small artery at the bottom centre of
the field in **320** shows thrombosis. **321** is a
section from the same field, which has been
stained to show elastin in black and collagen in
red. Disruption of the elastic layers and wall of
the artery are seen. The same vessel is shown at
higher magnification in **322**. It has been stained
by the MSB technique to show fibrin in red.
There is inflammatory destruction of the wall of
the artery, and fibrinoid material within its
lumen. This inflammatory, fibrinoid necrosis of
small arteries is typical of polyarteritis nodosa.

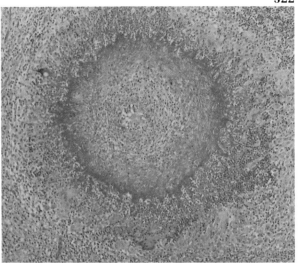
322

323 **Obscure gastrointestinal bleeding.**
Bleeding from the small or large intestine can
cause major diagnostic and management
problems. Clues to the likely aetiology of
bleeding may be apparent on physical
examination. The association of hereditary
haemorrhagic telangiectasia and gastrointestinal
bleeding is illustrated in **10** and **11**. This
photograph is of an elderly woman with
multiple haemangiomas of the tongue and
gastrointestinal tract.

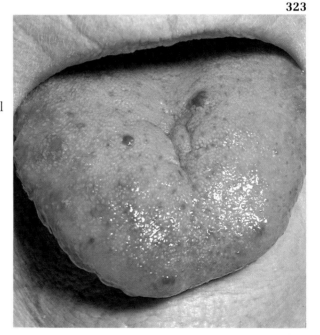
323

324 **Obscure gastrointestinal bleeding.** This is a
colonoscopic view of the transverse colon of a patient
who had presented on the previous day with the passage
of a large amount of dark blood clot and melaena per
rectum. Patches of jet black melaena stool are visible in
the transverse colon. No cause for the haemorrhage was
found at colonoscopy. The presence of melaena usually
suggests that the source of the bleeding is proximal to the
colon.

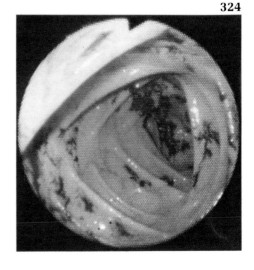
324

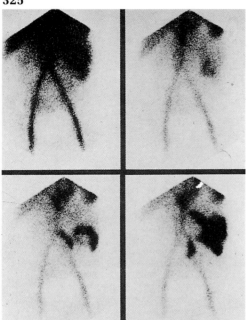

325 Obscure gastrointestinal bleeding. If a patient presents with an acute bleed, then upper gastrointestinal endoscopy or colonoscopy, or both, should be performed early whenever possible. If no cause is apparent, and the patient is still thought to be bleeding, angiography should be considered. **319** shows the angiographic appearance of a patient bleeding into the caecum from polyarteritis nodosa. If a bleeding site is not found on angiography, but slow or intermittent bleeding is continuing, a technetium-labelled red blood cell scan may be valuable in locating the source. In this case the upper right scan shows technetium-labelled red cells pooling in the upper jejunum. The lower scans were performed later in the study, and confirm that the labelled red cells have progressed into more-distal loops of small intestine.

326

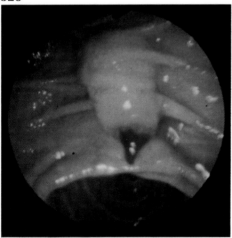

326 Haemobilia is a rare cause of obscure gastrointestinal bleeding. This endoscopic view shows a blood clot protruding from the ampulla of Vater into the second part of the duodenum in a patient who had passed a melaena stool. Haemobilia usually follows abdominal trauma, surgical treatment of biliary disease, or liver biopsy. Occasionally it may result from bleeding aneurysms or vascular tumours within the liver.

327

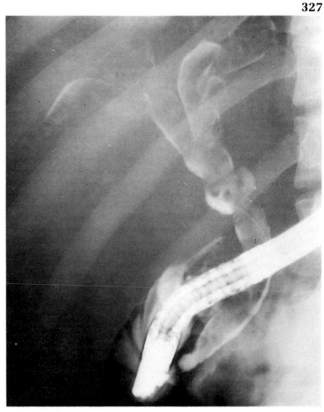

327 Haemobilia. An endoscopic retrograde cholangiogram demonstrating the presence of blood clot within the biliary tree (with contrast passing around the clot). This patient had bled from a tiny aneurysm within the right lobe of the liver. Treatment was by embolisation of the aneurysm.

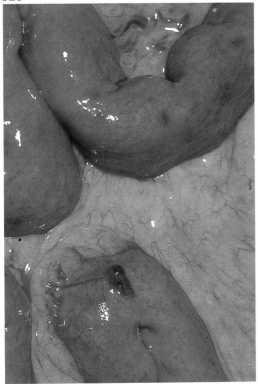

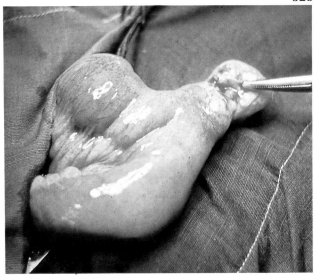

329 Meckel's diverticulum. This solitary diverticulum of the terminal ileum occurs in about 2% of the population. Symptoms are unusual, but haemorrhage, perforation or diverticulitis may occur. Symptoms usually occur in children or young adults. These complications are often due to acid secretion by ectopic gastric epithelium within the diverticulum, which causes peptic ulceration of the mucosa of either the diverticulum or the adjacent ileum. In this case the diverticulum has ulcerated and perforated, causing generalised peritonitis. The diverticulum and a portion of adjacent ileum was resected, and end-to-end anastomosis was performed.

328 Vascular malformations of the small intestine. A variety of arterial, venous or capillary malformations may be found in the gastrointestinal tract. This view at laparotomy demonstrates multiple venous ectasias of the small intestine.

330 Meckel's diverticulum, identified by means of a ^{99}Tc pertechnetate scan. The isotope has accumulated within the ectopic gastric mucosa, resulting in a focal area of uptake within the central abdomen (arrow) (compare with **178**).

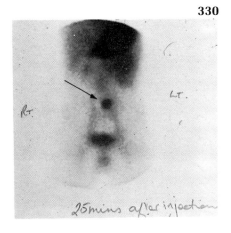

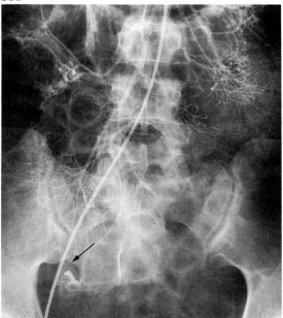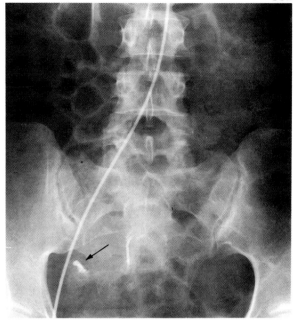

331 and **332**   **Meckel's diverticulum.** This is a superior mesenteric arteriogram in a young woman who presented with recurrent episodes of the passage of dark red blood per rectum. **331** is a film of early filling, showing a blush in the superior mesenteric arterial vasculature. Bleeding into a Meckel's diverticulum is demonstrated in the right iliac fossa (arrow). **332** is a later film: contrast is still pooled within the diverticulum, proving that this was the site of the bleeding (arrow). Patients with bleeding Meckel's diverticula often give a previous history of episodes of unexplained gastrointestinal haemorrhage over many years.

333

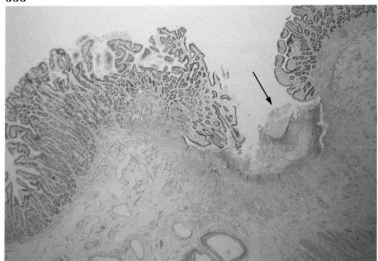

333   **Meckel's diverticulum.** The mucosa on the left is of gastric body type. That on the right is of small bowel type, more usual at this site. In between there is a benign peptic ulcer (arrow).

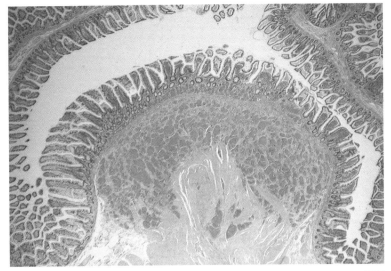

334 Meckel's diverticulum.
A carcinoid tumour is seen within the tip of this diverticulum in the centre of the field—a not uncommon association. The carcinoid is covered by mucosa of small intestinal type.

335 Jejunal carcinoma. Small intestinal neoplasms are rare. Although the small bowel provides about 80% of the luminal surface area of the entire alimentary canal, less than 2% of alimentary cancers develop here. Carcinoma of the jejunum usually presents with subacute intestinal obstruction or chronic intestinal blood loss, or both, as the tumour tends to be annular and ulcerated. Carcinomas of the ileum usually occur in association with Crohn's disease or Meckel's diverticulum. This barium follow-through examination was performed in an elderly woman with recurrent episodes of melaena. An annular carcinoma of the upper jejunum is demonstrated (arrows).

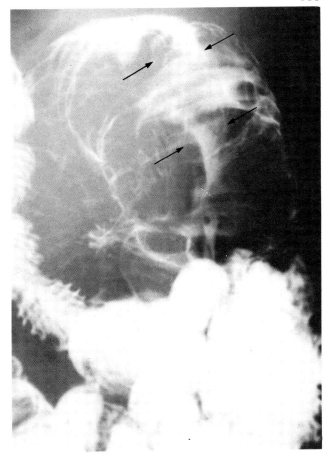

336

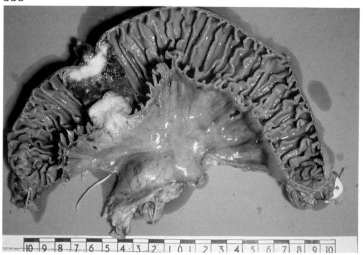

336 Jejunal carcinoma. This is a resection specimen showing an annular constricting jejunal carcinoma.

337

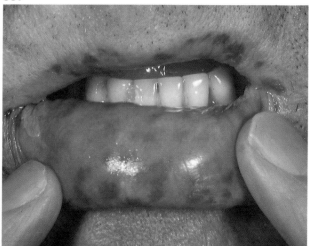

337 Peutz–Jeghers syndrome is a dominantly inherited disorder characterised by mucocutaneous pigmentation and gastrointestinal polyposis. Peutz–Jeghers polyps may occur anywhere in the intestine and may become malignant. The photograph shows the characteristic circumoral pigmentation of the syndrome. The pigmentation may not be as obvious as in this patient, and it should always be sought carefully in young patients presenting with unexplained gastrointestinal bleeding, particularly if there is a family history of such bleeding.

338

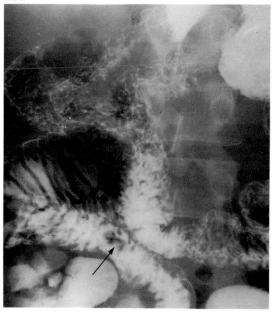

338 Peutz–Jeghers syndrome. This is a barium follow-through examination in a young adult with Peutz–Jeghers syndrome. Multiple polyps have given rise to a coarsened mucosal pattern in the upper small intestinal loop, and larger filling defects are seen in the ileum (arrow).

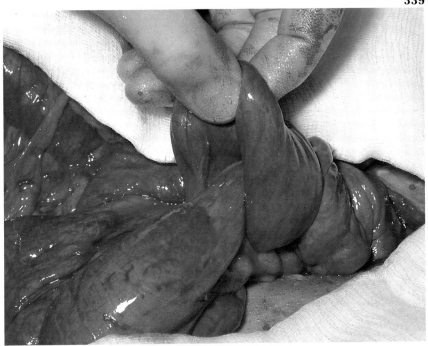

339   Peutz–Jeghers syndrome. An operative view of the same patient as in **338**, taken earlier in the course of his illness. Intussusception of a jejunal polyp has occurred, giving rise to jejunal obstruction. Gastrointestinal bleeding and malignancy are the other characteristic complications of Peutz–Jeghers polyps. Prophylactic resection of small intestine may be indicated if polyps larger than 1 cm in diameter are discovered on x-ray examination, because of the risk of intussusception and subsequent infarction of small intestine. Some patients with Peutz–Jeghers syndrome have suffered many complications necessitating repeated small intestinal resections, leading to a shortened bowel syndrome.

340   Peutz–Jeghers syndrome. An hamartomatous polyp from the jejunum of a patient with Peutz–Jeghers syndrome. These polyps contain a branching core and are covered by non-neoplastic small intestinal epithelium.

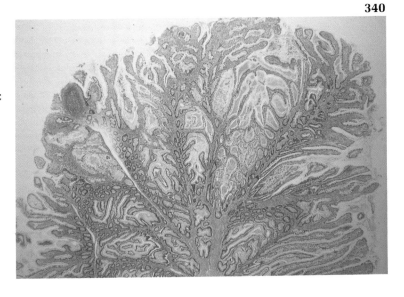

341

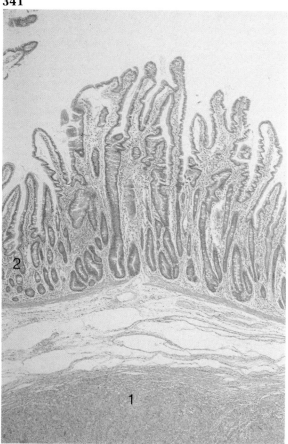

341 Peutz–Jeghers syndrome. The same patient as **340**, showing a very early stage in the formation of a polyp in addition to a focus of small bowel adenocarcinoma (1). The mucosa on the left is almost normal (2). The exaggerated mucosa of the incipient polyp is seen at the centre of the picture.

342

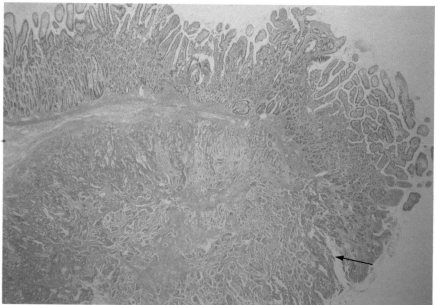

342 Peutz–Jeghers syndrome. Patients with Peutz–Jeghers polyposis have an increased risk, albeit small, of gastrointestinal carcinoma. This patient developed poorly differentiated carcinoma of the small bowel (arrow). There is an abrupt change between carcinoma and normal mucosa in the upper part of the field.

343 Secondary tumour deposits in the intestine. A small bowel biopsy of a patient with disseminated carcinoma of the breast. Two villi contain poorly differentiated adenocarcinoma (arrows). The remainder of the mucosa is a little inflamed.

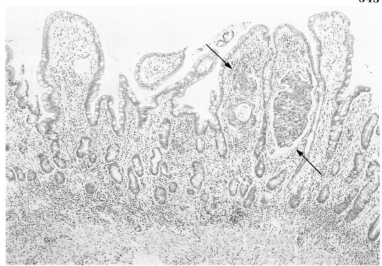

344 Secondary melanoma deposits in the intestine. Metastatic melanoma deposits in the small or large intestine are found at autopsy in about half of the patients dying of disseminated disease. Patients with disseminated melanoma do not usually survive sufficiently long to develop complications from intestinal secondary deposits, but occasionally operation becomes necessary for intestinal obstruction, bleeding or perforation. The figure shows multiple secondary deposits of melanoma in the colon.

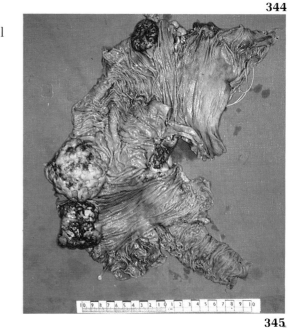

345 Secondary melanoma deposits in the intestine. A duodenal biopsy from a patient with melanoma. The tip of a villus is seen at high magnification. It contains many malignant cells, some of which contain a little pigment.

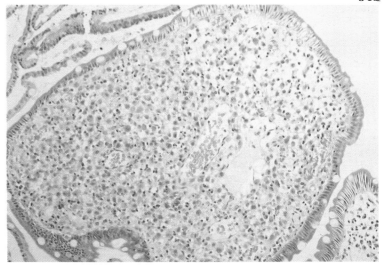

346

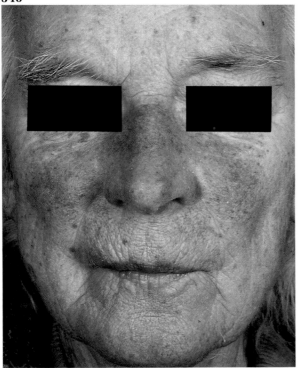

346 Carcinoid syndrome. This rare syndrome results from a malignant tumour of the enterochromaffin cells of the intestine (usually the jejunum or ileum) with secondary deposits in the liver. Typically the liver deposits become massive, and they secrete a variety of vasoactive substances into the blood stream, especially 5-hydroxytryptamine (5-HT). Flushing and diarrhoea are the characteristic clinical presentations of this syndrome. The flushing may be paroxysmal, precipitated by alcohol or certain foods. Patients with recurrent facial flushing may develop a violaceous discolouration of the skin with telangiectasia, as in this patient.

347

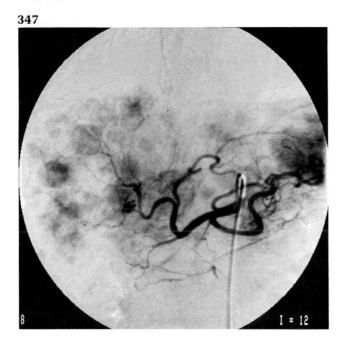

347 Carcinoid syndrome. A digital subtraction selective hepatic arteriogram, demonstrating multiple tumour blushes within the liver substance. Following this angiogram, hepatic arterial embolisation was carried out in an attempt to control the flushing and diarrhoea that had developed in this patient. Very worthwhile responses may result from tumour embolisation, which is safer than surgical resection for the palliation of symptoms. The other indication for hepatic embolisation in carcinoid syndrome is relief of pain from rapidly enlarging hepatic secondary deposits. A variety of drugs that prevent the synthesis or antagonise the peripheral effects of 5-HT have been tried, including methysergide and cyproheptadine. Many patients with carcinoid syndrome have survived for more than 10 years despite a high tumour load. For this reason the palliation of symptoms is very worthwhile.

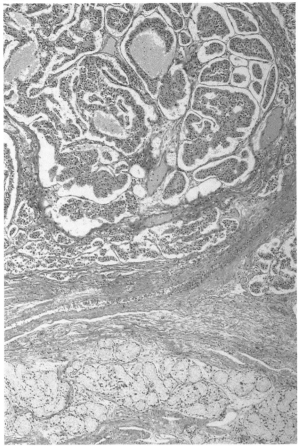

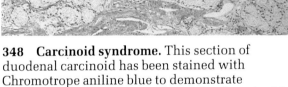

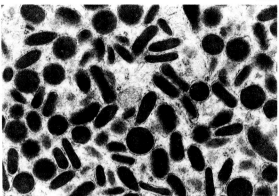

349 Carcinoid syndrome. Carcinoid tumours of the small intestine are usually found to contain dense, pleomorphic, membrane-bound granules containing 5-HT, as shown here on electron microscopy (orig. mag. × 22,500).

348 Carcinoid syndrome. This section of duodenal carcinoid has been stained with Chromotrope aniline blue to demonstrate connective tissue. Nests and islands of carcinoid tumour cells are seen above, and there is a Brunner's gland below.

350 Pellagra. This photosensitive eruption occurs as a result of nicotinic acid deficiency. In white skins there may be prominent sebaceous follicles of the nose and a red or dusky brown well-circumscribed dermatitis. In dark skins the lesions are relatively depigmented and scaly, as in this example. Nicotinic acid deficiency may give rise to dementia and diarrhoea, and is uncommon in Western civilisations. Disturbed tryptophan metabolism may give rise to pellagra in patients with the carcinoid syndrome.

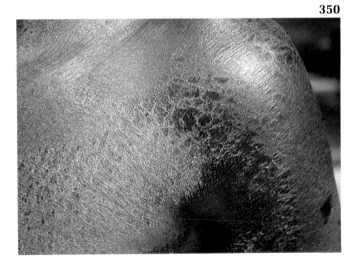

351

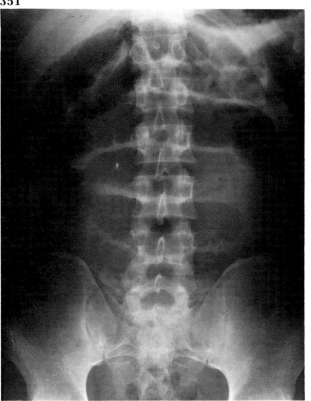

351 Small intestinal obstruction commonly arises from a strangulated femoral or inguinal hernia (see Chapter 9). Other causes include a carcinoma of the caecum, Crohn's disease of the terminal ileum, adhesions and gallstone ileus. The characteristic symptoms are colicky abdominal pain, effortless vomiting (which may be faeculent) absolute constipation and abdominal distension. This plain supine abdominal x-ray was from a patient with low small intestinal obstruction due to lymphoma. The distended small bowel loops occupy most of the abdominal cavity, giving rise to this so-called step-ladder pattern.

352

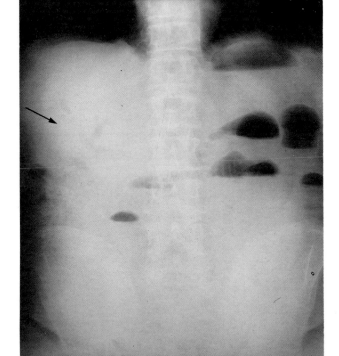

352 Small intestinal obstruction. This is a plain abdominal x-ray of a patient with small bowel obstruction, taken with the patient in an erect position. Multiple fluid levels are seen within dilated loops of small intestine. In this particular case the cause was a gallstone ileus. Air is visible within the biliary tree (arrow).

CHAPTER 9

Hernias

353 Inguinal hernia. An inguinal hernia is the protrusion of peritoneal contents into the inguinal canal. The most common variety is the indirect inguinal hernia which enters the canal via the internal inguinal ring. Direct inguinal hernias penetrate forward through the posterior wall of the inguinal canal. These two types of inguinal hernia may be difficult to distinguish clinically. Indirect inguinal hernias are commonly bilateral. Inguinal hernias are usually reducible. Operation is usually advised. Inguinal herniorrhaphy consists of excision of the hernial sac and repair of the weakened inguinal canal. Direct inguinal hernias are much more likely to recur after repair than are indirect hernias.

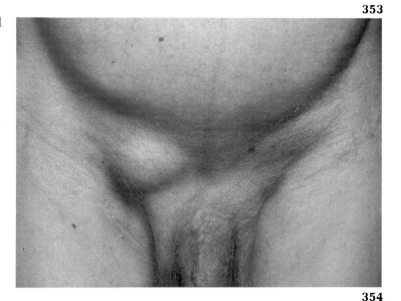

354 Scrotal hernia. Large indirect inguinal hernias pass through the internal inguinal ring, down the inguinal canal as far as the external ring and into the neck of the scrotum. In this example a huge inguinal hernia has become incarcerated within the scrotal compartment. A para-umbilical hernia is also present in this man with ascites.

355

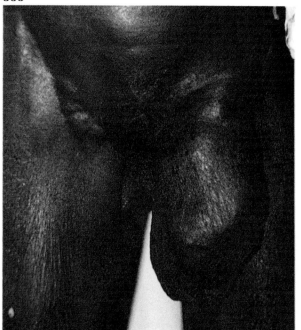

355 Femoral hernia arises from the protrusion of peritoneal contents through the femoral canal. They may be distinguished clinically from inguinal hernias as they are located below and lateral to the pubic tubercle. Femoral hernias occur more commonly in females than in males, because of the wider female pelvis. Irreducibility and strangulation are common complications of femoral hernia because the femoral canal is narrow. For this reason all femoral hernias should be repaired by excision of the sac and closure of the femoral canal.

356

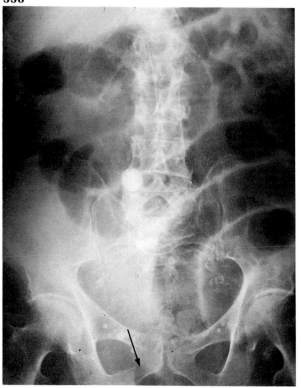

356 Small bowel obstruction due to hernia. Part of the small intestine may become trapped within the hernial sac. Small intestinal obstruction or strangulation, or both, may result. A tender, tense, irreducible hernia may be palpable in the inguinal or femoral canal. Strangulated hernia is the most common cause of small bowel obstruction. The dilated, obstructed small bowel loops are seen on this plain abdominal x-ray; there is gas within the strangulated small bowel loop seen outside the peritoneal cavity (arrow). At operation the bowel is congested and may be gangrenous. In cases of doubtful viability it is wise to perform a small bowel resection and end-to-end anastomosis.

357 Strangulated inguinal hernia.
This resection specimen from a patient
with a strangulated inguinal hernia
illustrates the gangrenous loop of small
bowel that had been trapped within the
hernial sac.

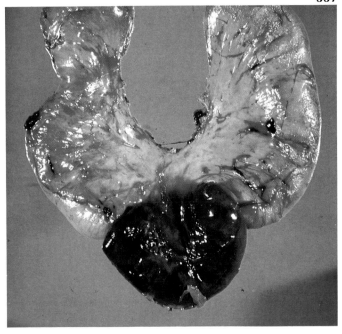

358 Strangulated hernia. Histological
examination of the strangulated small intestine
from the specimen in **357** demonstrates gross
mucosal and submucosal oedema, congestion
and extravasation of red cells.

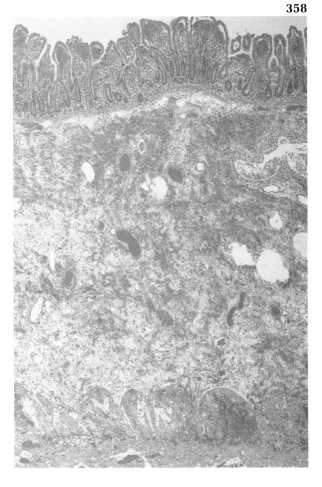

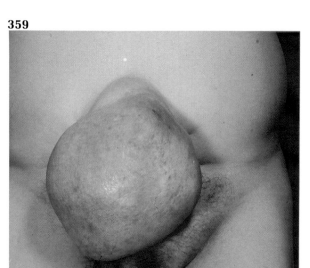

359 Para-umbilical hernia. This type of hernia may occur just above or below the umbilicus. It is commonly seen in patients with obesity or ascites, usually contains omentum and may contain portions of transverse colon or small intestine, or both. Operative reduction is normally advised. If the patient has ascites, then attention should be given to the underlying cause.

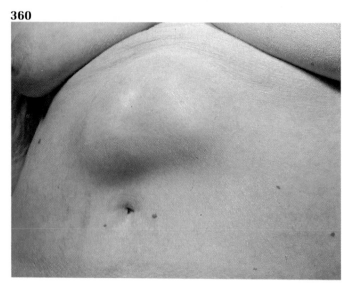

360 Ventral hernia. A midline ventral hernia may occur as an elongated gap between the recti, and is common in older patients. The elderly woman in the figure had ascites secondary to chronic active hepatitis and cirrhosis, as well as a ventral hernia.

CHAPTER 10

The Normal Colon and Rectum

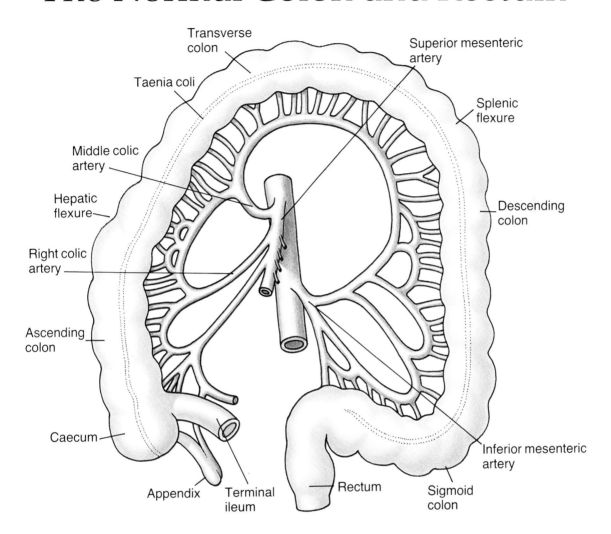

This structure travels three sides of a square from the right iliac fossa to the left side of the pelvis. It then follows a tortuous course in the pelvis and forms a reservoir, the rectum. Sensation of faecal matter in the rectum usually results in the desire to defecate.

The appendix is a worm-shaped structure, with a blind terminal, that opens into the caecum. Its position is notoriously variable.

The caecum is a blind cul-de-sac situated below the ileocaecal orifice. The ascending colon lies posteriorly in the right side of the abdomen, and is related to the iliac crest. The hepatic flexure is a sharp bend situated below the right lobe of the liver and in front of the right kidney. The transverse colon is suspended on a long mesentery, and lies anterior to the second part of the duodenum and the greater curve of the stomach. The colon turns posteriorly again at the splenic flexure, so that the descending colon is held down by a layer of peritoneum. The sigmoid colon lies on a mesentery and is variable in length.

The colon acts as a reservoir for the ileal

effluent, and is responsible for the absorption of water and electrolytes and, to a lesser extent, the secretion of electrolytes. Its luminal surface is lined by mucus-secreting columnar epithelium. Like the small intestine, there are inner circular and outer longitudinal muscle coats; the longitudinal is arranged in three narrow bands, the taeniae coli.

The right colon and the proximal two-thirds of the transverse colon derive the bulk of their blood supply from the right and middle colic arteries, which are branches of the superior mesenteric artery. The left colon and rectum are supplied by branches of the inferior mesenteric artery. There is an anastomosis between the superior and inferior mesenteric arterial trees within the transverse mesentery. The rectum is supplied by three pairs of rectal arteries which arise from the internal iliac arteries. Venous drainage occurs via the superior and inferior mesenteric veins, and thence into the portal vein.

The ano-rectum is a site of porto-systemic anastomosis, so that haemorrhoidal varices may develop if portal hypertension is present. The autonomic nerve supply to the colon follows the distribution of the arterial supply, such that vagal parasympathetic fibres arise from the coeliac plexus, and pelvic splanchnic nerves ascend from the pelvic parasympathetic outflow. Sympathetic connections arise from the abdominal paraganglia. The pelvic splanchnic nerves also carry afferent fibres (sensitive to pain and distension), from the rectum above the anal canal.

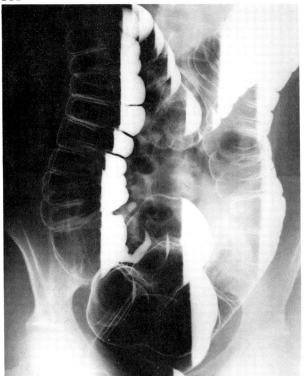

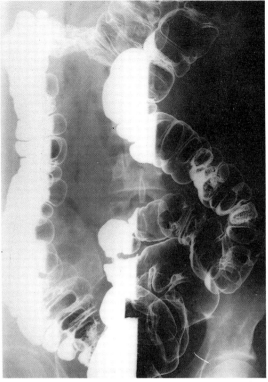

361 Normal barium enema. Double-contrast barium studies of the colon are commonly performed early in the course of investigations for patients with large bowel symptoms. Barium and air are introduced via a rectal catheter into the whole length of the prepared colon. Single-contrast barium enemas will fail to provide the mucosal detail that is seen in this x-ray, and may miss important mucosal lesions. This double-contrast barium enema film was taken with the patient lying in the left decubitus position, allowing detailed visualisation of the caecum and ascending colon. The appendix is commonly filled, as in this x-ray. Reflux of barium into the terminal ileum may provide further important information, particularly in patients with suspected Crohn's disease.

362 Normal barium enema. The shape of the colon is often tortuous, as in this patient. It may prove impossible to identify abnormalities in the overlapping loops of sigmoid colon. Another potential mistake is to miss the splenic flexure (as in this x-ray).

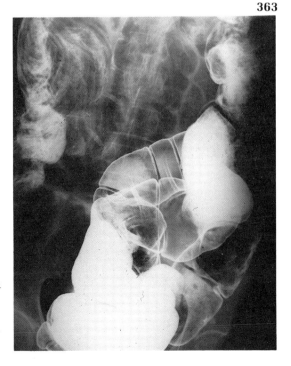

363 Barium enema — poor preparation. Vigorous cleansing of the bowel is necessary before barium enema. Patients are usually encouraged to adhere to a low-fibre diet and to take laxatives before the examination. Rectal washouts may also be necessary. Failure to prepare the bowel may result in an unsatisfactory examination, due to faeces still in the colonic lumen, as in this example. Occasionally an instant enema (without preparation) is performed in patients with ulcerative colitis.

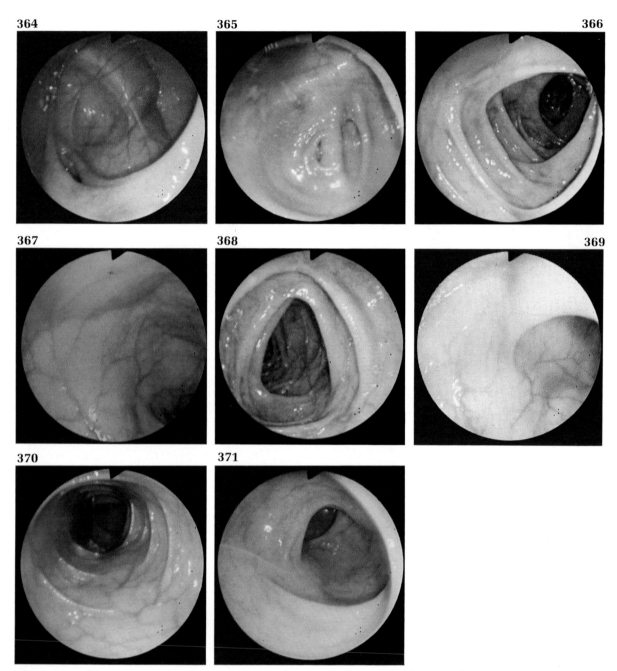

364 to 371   Normal colonoscopy. 364 shows the appearance of the ileocaecal valve shortly after withdrawal of the instrument from the terminal ileum. Experienced colonoscopists can enter the terminal ileum in up to 75% of patients. The normal appearance of the caecum with its triradiate fold and appendiceal orifice are seen in **365**. Some small bowel effluent is usually present in the caecum, as in the top part of the photograph. The rounded triangular haustral folds of the ascending colon are seen in **366**. **367** is a close-up view of the hepatic flexure region, illustrating the bluish appearance from the adjacent right lobe of liver. The normal colonic vasculature is demonstrated clearly. The sharp triangular folds of the transverse colon are shown in **368**. This section lies in the abdomen suspended by the transverse mesocolon. Consequently, the transverse colon is very mobile and may be difficult to examine with the colonoscope. **369** shows bluish indentation of the spleen, with the instrument withdrawn to the splenic flexure. The descending colon is shown in **370**. This is the narrowest part of the colon. It is fixed by peritoneum anteriorly and on both sides by the paracolic gutter. For this reason it is usually an easy part of the colon to examine, and it appears as a long, fixed tunnel with a more rounded haustral pattern than is seen in the right colon. **371** is a view of the sigmoid colon. This part of the colon lies on a triangular mesentry and is often tortuous.

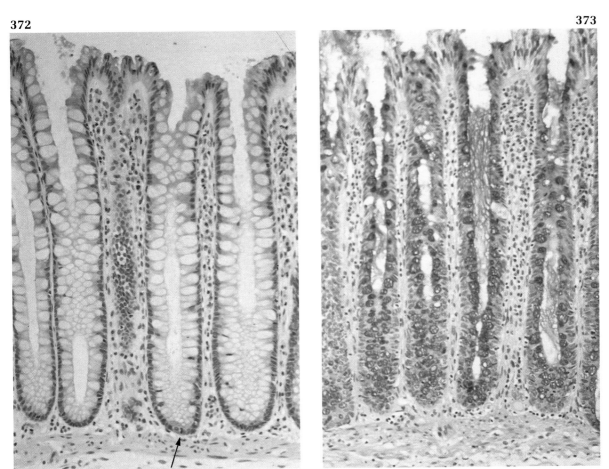

372 and **373**   **Normal large bowel mucosa.** The glands are simple and straight. The crypt bases rest on the muscularis mucosa, and the one in the centre of **372** contains a red-staining enteroendocrine cell (arrow). The lamina propria consists of a little connective tissue with a few lymphocytes and plasma cells. **373** is a similar preparation stained with alcian blue–diastase PAS to demonstrate mucin. Normal large bowel epithelium produces acid mucus only, as seen here.

374

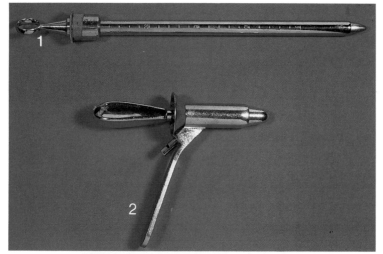

375

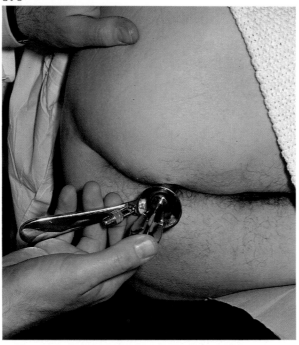

374 and 375   Proctoscopy and sigmoidoscopy. The rigid instruments that are used routinely in outpatients departments for the examination of the rectum and recto-sigmoid regions are shown in **374**. They are inserted with the patient lying on the left side, as in **375**. After insertion of each instrument, the internal obturator is removed and a fibreoptic light source is connected. The rigid sigmoidoscope ((1) in **374**) is usually 20–30 cm in length. The proctoscope ((2) in **374**, and **375**) is normally used for the investigation of low rectal or anal conditions, such as haemorrhoids.

376

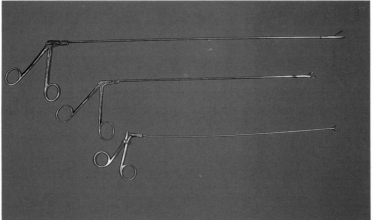

376   Rectal biopsy forceps. A variety of different mucosal biopsy forceps are shown. Note the different size of the 'bites'. The forceps are introduced into the rectum or recto-sigmoid via the rigid sigmoidoscope, and allow a small fragment of mucosa to be grasped and removed for histology. Rectal mucosal biopsy is performed for the histological confirmation of carcinomas, and in the diagnosis and assessment of inflammatory bowel disease.

377 to 379   Flexible sigmoidoscopy. This technique is becoming more widely used in outpatient clinics for the investigation of rectal bleeding and altered bowel habit. The flexible sigmoidoscope (**377**) can often be negotiated throughout the rectum and sigmoid colon, covering the area where more than half of colonic tumours arise. The typical accompanying light-source assembly is shown on a trolley in **378**. Facilities are available for mucosal biopsy (**379**), suction and even polypectomy using a snare diathermy technique.

377

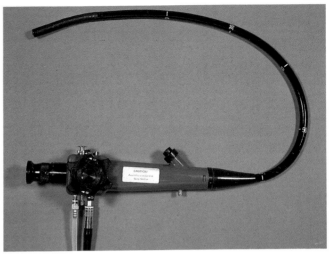

378

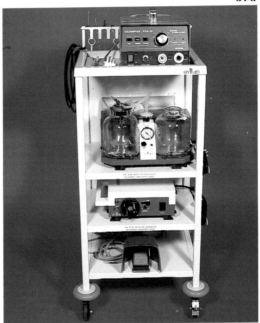

379

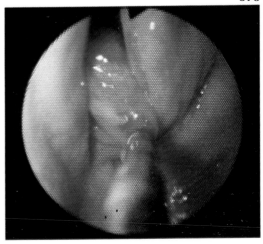

CHAPTER 11

Diseases of the Colon and Rectum

380

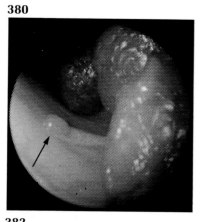

381

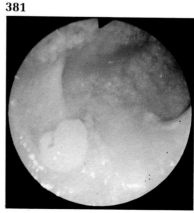

380 and **381   Metaplastic polyps.** This is the most common variety of polyp found in the colon. Up to 75% of adults over the age of 40 years have metaplastic polyps. **380** is a colonoscopic view of a poorly prepared bowel (the large masses are faeces) and a tiny sessile metaplastic polyp on a haustral fold (arrow). A larger example is shown in **381**. The risk of malignant transformation in metaplastic polyps is very low.

382

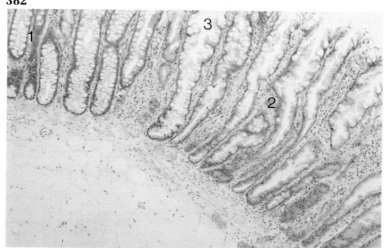

382   Metaplastic polyps. The normal rectal mucosa is seen to the left of the field (1) and the metaplastic polyp lies to the right (2). The mucosa of the polyp is taller than normal and has a curious fibrillated epithelial contour (3).

383

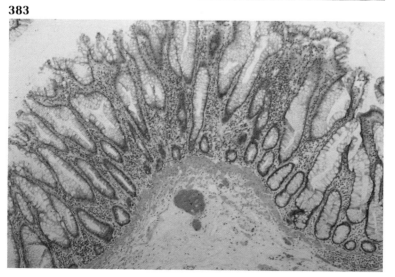

383   Metaplastic polyps. This section illustrates a further phase in the evolution of the polyp. As it enlarges, its base is drawn towards the luminal surface. The mucosa of the polyp is hyperplastic and shows the typical superficial epithelial serration.

384 Inflammatory polyps are most commonly seen in patients with ulcerative colitis (see **503**). This is the histological appearance of an inflammatory polyp from the rectum of a patient with ulcerative colitis. The polyp consists of inflamed granulation tissue covered by inflammatory debris. Inflamed mucosa is seen to either side of its base.

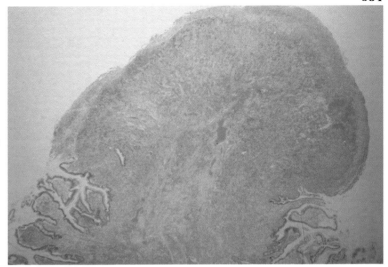

385 Inflammatory polyps evolve into regenerative polyps when the inflammation has subsided. A small focus of ulceration remains at the upper left of this section, where inflamed granulation tissue is seen. The regenerative epithelium still shows architectural disturbance; presumably this abnormality would have resolved had healing been allowed to proceed to completion.

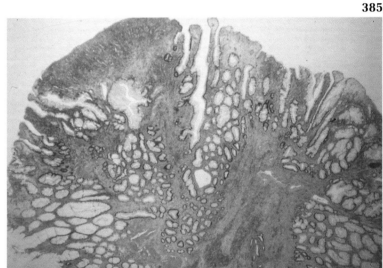

386 Villous adenoma.
An operative resection specimen from an elderly man with a large caecal villous adenoma. Patients with villous adenomas may present with diarrhoea due to excessive mucus production, which may even lead to fluid, protein and electrolyte loss. Occasionally they may intussuscept, causing abdominal discomfort or intestinal obstruction. Large villous adenomas commonly undergo malignant transformation.

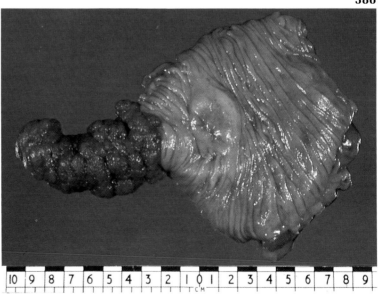

387

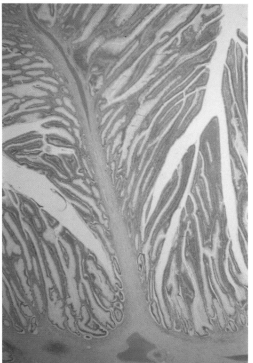

387 Villous adenoma. A section of a rectal polyp. The neoplastic epithelium forms papillary processes to either side of the central polyp base. The adenomatous process may involve large areas of the rectal mucosa.

388

389

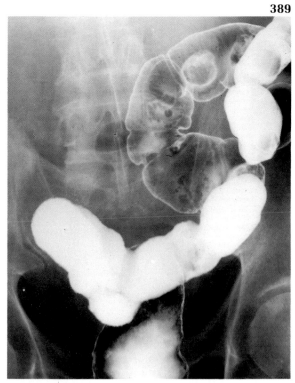

388 and 389 Adenomatous polyps. Barium enema is usually performed after sigmoidoscopy for the investigation of rectal bleeding. A pedunculated polyp 1 cm in diameter is shown in **388** (arrow). Meticulous double-contrast technique is required for the identification of colonic polyps—the colon must be well prepared and completely clear of all faecal residue. **389** illustrates a diagnostic pitfall that may result from poor preparation: retained lumps of faeces in the sigmoid colon makes interpretation difficult. A pedunculated polyp 3 cm in diameter was later identified at colonoscopy.

390 Adenomatous polyps. A large polyp on a long stalk has been identified in the sigmoid colon at colonoscopy in an elderly man presenting with rectal bleeding. Bleeding is thought to result from trauma due to peristaltic waves and contact with overlying faeces. The mucosa covering the polyp is friable and haemorrhagic. The risk of malignant transformation in an adenomatous polyp increases with the size of the polyp. The identification of a polyp by sigmoidoscopy or barium enema is an indication for a full-length colonoscopy to exclude other polyps or carcinomas. Furthermore, colonoscopy provides an opportunity for removal of any polyps by hot biopsy or snare technique (see **391** to **394**).

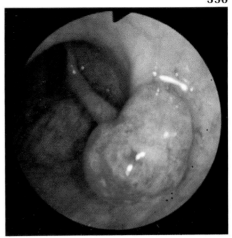

390

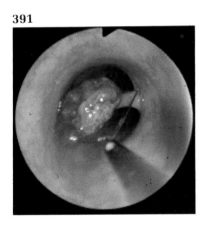

391

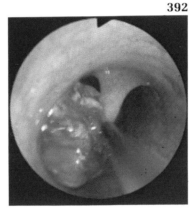

392

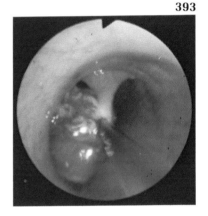

393

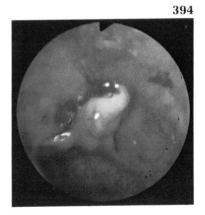

394

391 to 394 Colonoscopic polypectomy. This technique is widely used for the removal of pedunculated (and some sessile) polyps during colonoscopy. A lasso-shaped snare within an insulated sheath is passed through the biopsy channel of the colonoscope towards the polyp. The snare is then opened (**391**), manoeuvred over the head of the polyp and gently closed to ensnare the stalk (**392**). Short bursts of current are applied via the diathermy snare to coagulate the blood vessels within the polyp in order to minimise bleeding. **393** illustrates the coagulation burns to part of the stalk and the cyanosed appearance of the polyp after electrocautery. Increasing amounts of current are applied for a few seconds at a time until the polyp has been removed. The snare is used to grasp the polyp so that it can be removed for histological examination. **394** shows the appearance of the remaining stalk with only slight bleeding following the procedure.

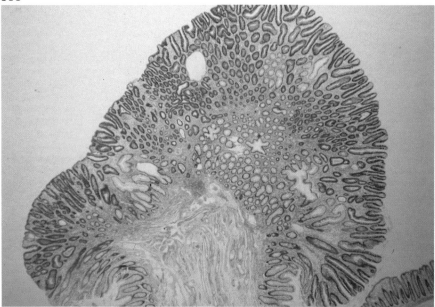

395 Adenomatous polyps. The histological spectrum of adenomatous polyps ranges from the villous (papillary) adenoma (**387**) to the tubular adenoma seen here, where the neoplastic epithelium has formed glands rather than villi. The epithelium covering the polyp is dysplastic and stains more darkly than the normal epithelium, which covers each side of the stalk at the bottom of the figure.

396

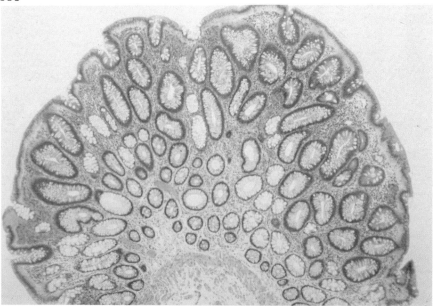

396 Adenomatous polyps. The darkly staining neoplastic epithelium of this tubular adenoma shows a slight degree of dysplasia only. Normal glandular epithelium is seen at the bottom. Colorectal adenomas are currently defined as epithelial neoplasms confined to the mucosa. The intact muscularis mucosa is seen here as the pink semicircle at the bottom centre of the field. Malignant transformation in an adenomatous polyp cannot be excluded unless the submucosa is shown to be free from infiltration.

397 Colonic polyposis. A photograph of a resected colon containing multiple small adenomatous polyps. One of these had undergone malignant change (arrow). Adenomatous polyps show dysplasia of their surface epithelium when they are examined histologically. It is believed that a small percentage of such polyps will undergo changes amounting to 'carcinoma-*in-situ*', and a proportion of these develop into invasive adenocarcinoma. Approximately 20% of patients with colorectal cancer are found to have adenomatous polyps elsewhere in the colon, either at the time of diagnosis or afterwards. Many experts believe that annual colonoscopy for early detection and treatment of adenomatous polyps is indicated in patients who have undergone resection of a carcinoma.

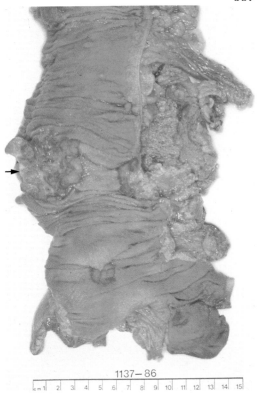

1137—86

398 Familial polyposis coli is the most common of the familial polyposis syndromes and is of autosomal dominant inheritance. The risk of carcinoma in patients with this syndrome approaches 100% by the age of 40 years. There are vast numbers of adenomatous polyps and a carcinoma in this resection specimen. Prophylactic colectomy and ileostomy is the standard treatment, but colectomy and ileorectal anastomosis with life-long sigmoidoscopic surveillance of the rectum is now being practised in some centres.

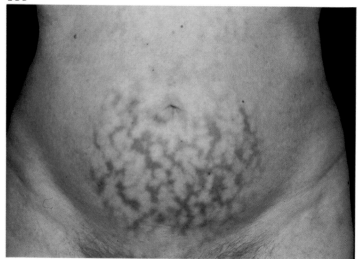

399 Erythema abigne. This localised rash develops in patients who apply hot-water bottles or other heat treatment to areas of pain. The presence of this rash in a patient presenting with abdominal pain strongly suggests an organic cause. This patient was found to have a carcinoma of the sigmoid colon on barium enema.

400

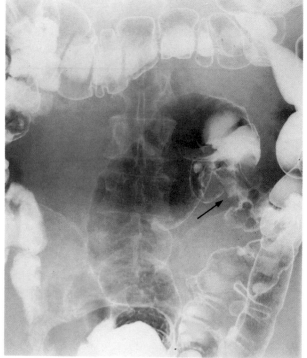

401

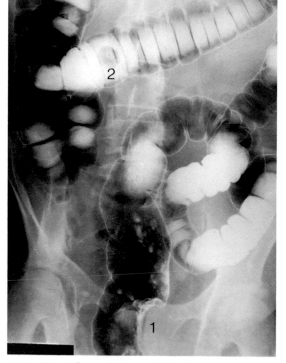

400 Colorectal carcinoma. Double-contrast barium enema is the standard method of making the diagnosis of colorectal carcinoma. This barium enema was performed in a patient with change of bowel habit and rectal bleeding. A malignant stricture has been identified in the sigmoid colon. It has the characteristic 'apple-core' appearance (arrow). The appearances are often not as typical as this, and in such cases it is wise to obtain histological confirmation by means of colonoscopy (or flexible sigmoidoscopy) and biopsy.

401 Rectal carcinoma. A barium enema showing a polypoid carcinoma of the rectum (1) that had been demonstrated on sigmoidoscopy. The barium enema was performed to exclude a synchronous polyp or carcinoma. A pedunculated polyp has been outlined in the proximal transverse colon (2). Rectal carcinomas can normally be resected and end-to-end anastomosis performed with the aid of a transrectal stapling gun. Low rectal tumours require abdominoperineal resection and the formation of a colostomy.

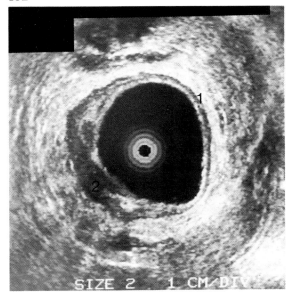

402 Rectal carcinoma. Transrectal ultrasound is being evaluated in the pre-operative assessment of the depth of invasion of rectal cancer. The inner circle in the centre of this image is the transducer. The large black space is the rectal lumen. The echogenic rectal mucosa and submucosa are separated by a rim of echo-poor (black) muscularis mucosa (1). Tumour has penetrated beyond the muscularis propria and serosa (2).

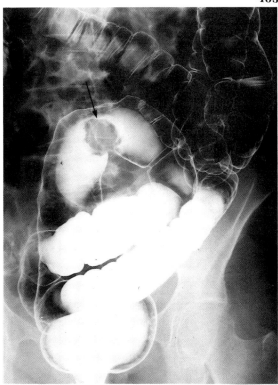

403 Colorectal carcinoma. Barium enema shows a large polypoid tumour in the sigmoid colon (arrow).

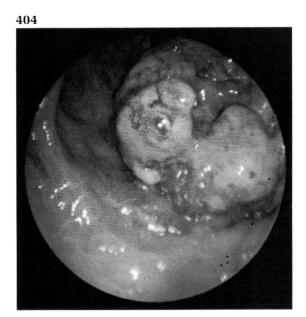

404 Colorectal carcinoma. An irregular polypoid carcinoma seen by colonoscopy.

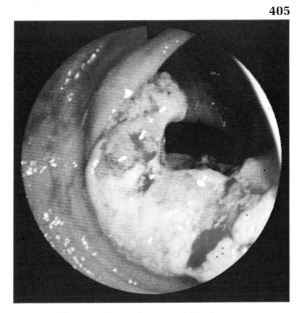

405 Colorectal carcinoma. This is a colonoscopic view of an annular carcinoma of the ascending colon. Carcinomas of the caecum and ascending colon commonly present with iron deficiency anaemia, as was the case in this patient.

406

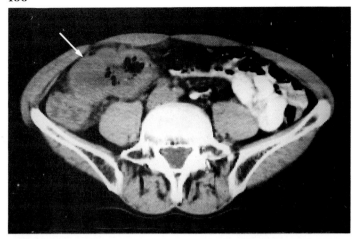

406 and **407**   **Colorectal carcinoma.**
Computerised tomography at two
different levels has been performed in
an elderly woman presenting with a
fixed mass in the right iliac fossa. A
locally invasive carcinoma of the
ascending colon is shown in **406**
(arrow). **407** is a higher cut
demonstrating a lymph node
metastasis below the hilum of the
liver (1). There is calcification in the
abdominal aorta (2). The right lobe of
the liver is free of secondary deposits.
Computerised tomography or
ultrasound are useful in the pre-
operative assessment of colorectal
carcinoma. However, a negative scan
does not exclude distant metastases.

407

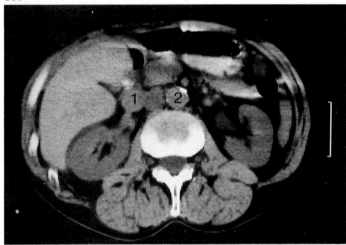

408

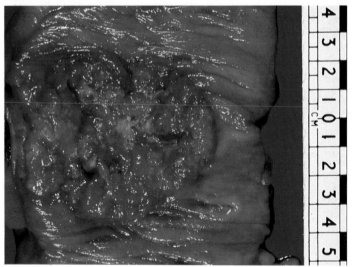

408   **Colorectal carcinoma.**
A colonic resection specimen from a
patient with a polypoid ulcerating
colonic carcinoma 6 cm in diameter.
Histological assessment of the
carcinoma and the mesenteric lymph
nodes is used to stage the tumour in
order to define prognosis. The Dukes
system is the most widely used
classification. Dukes' stage A
carcinomas are confined to the bowel
wall and carry a mean 5-year survival
of 85%. Tumours that have infiltrated
the whole thickness of the bowel wall,
in the absence of lymph node
metastases, are classified as stage B
and have a mean 65% 5-year survival
after resection. The prognosis
becomes worse once the regional
lymph nodes (especially the apical
mesenteric lymph node) are involved
(Dukes' stage C). The 5-year survival
in patients with untreated liver
metastases is less than 1%.

409 and **410** **Colorectal carcinoma. 409** is a section from the mucosal edge of a moderately differentiated adenocarcinoma of the colon. There is an abrupt transition between virtually normal glands at the right to a gland lined by neoplastic epithelium to the left of centre which is then continuous with the infiltrative carcinoma. A deeper section from the same carcinoma is seen at higher magnification in **410**. The carcinoma cells are hyperchromatic and pleomorphic with enlarged nuclei, prominent nucleoli, an increased nuclear/cytoplasmic ratio and plentiful mitosis. These are the cytological features of malignancy.

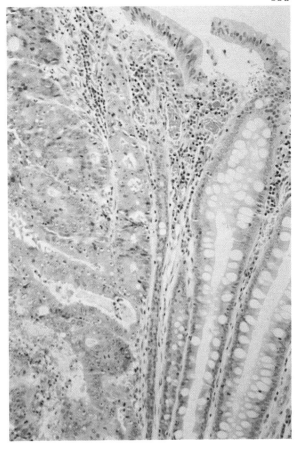

410

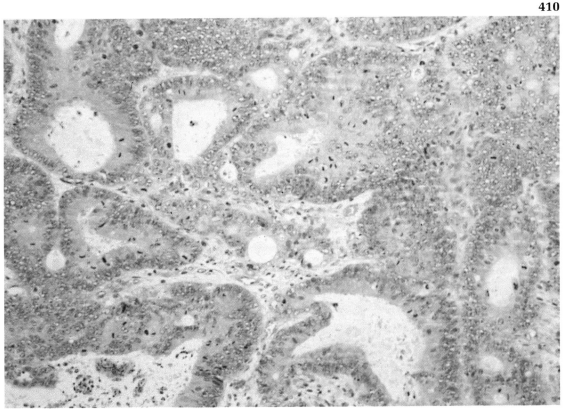

411

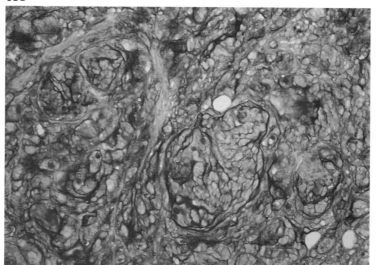

411 Colorectal carcinoma.
A mucoid (colloid) carcinoma of the
colon, stained for mucins with
alcian blue–diastase PAS.
Occasional tumour cells are hidden
in the abundant extracellular mucus.

412

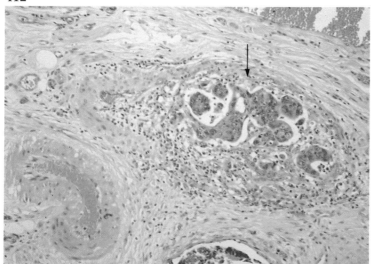

412 Colorectal carcinoma.
A submucosal vein at the edge of an
average grade adenocarcinoma of the
colon. Vascular invasion is seen
(arrow), and this is the first step in
the spread of such tumours to the
liver.

413

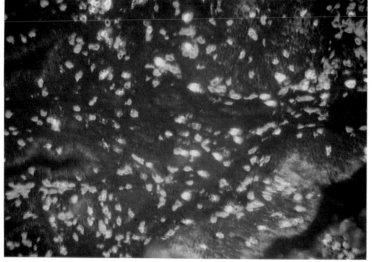

413 Colorectal carcinoma.
An immunofluorescence preparation
in a colonic biopsy with severe
mucosal dysplasia. The CD4
lymphocytes (helper-inducer subset)
appear green. There is marked
infiltration of the lamina propria
with T-lymphocytes of this subset.
This cell-mediated immune
response may play a role in
preventing the development of frank
invasive carcinoma.

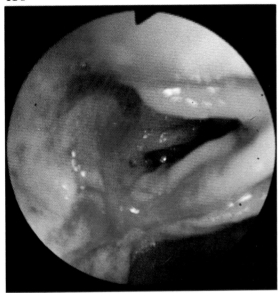

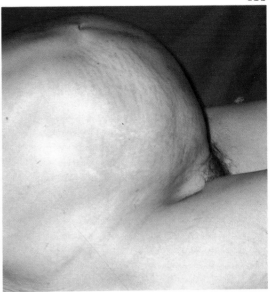

414   Colorectal carcinoma. A colonoscopic
view of a large ulcerating carcinoma of the
splenic flexure that has tethered and
compressed the colonic lumen. Surprisingly,
this tumour had not been identified on barium
enema. Histological examination of
colonoscopic biopsies confirmed the diagnosis.

415   Colorectal carcinoma. A photograph
of the abdomen of a patient with complete
large bowel obstruction due to a carcinoma
of the sigmoid colon. The symptoms were
colicky lower abdominal pain, gross
abdominal distension and absolute
constipation (no faeces or flatus for the
previous 4 days). Auscultation of the
abdomen revealed hyperactive, tinkling
bowel sounds. Other causes of complete
large bowel obstruction include sigmoid
volvulus, external herniae and faecal
impaction.

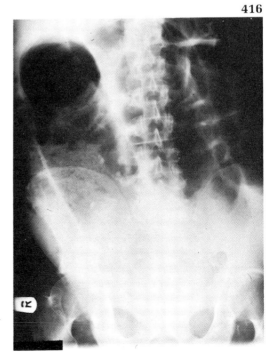

416   Colorectal carcinoma. A supine plain abdominal
x-ray from a patient with colonic obstruction due to a
sigmoid carcinoma.

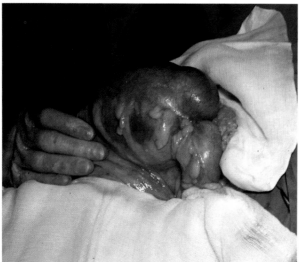

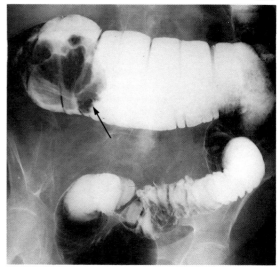

417   Colorectal carcinoma. An operative photograph of colonic obstruction due to a carcinoma. The usual surgical approach in cases such as this is to resect the carcinoma and bring out the obstructed loop as a colostomy. The colostomy is closed and end-to-end anastomosis performed when the patient's condition has improved.

418   Colorectal carcinoma. Intussusception of a polypoid colorectal carcinoma is an unusual complication. This barium enema has outlined a polypoid caecal carcinoma (arrow) that has intussuscepted into the proximal transverse colon. Other emergency complications of colorectal carcinoma include intestinal obstruction, haemorrhage and perforation.

419

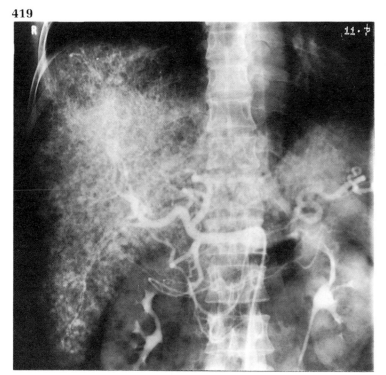

419   Colorectal carcinoma. A hepatic arteriogram demonstrating multiple tumour blushes within the liver in a patient with metastases due to colorectal carcinoma. Computerised tomography or ultrasound are preferred to angiography for the diagnosis of liver metastases. Arteriography is occasionally performed before embolisation of painful liver metastases. Unfortunately, metastatic spread from colorectal carcinoma responds poorly to chemotherapy. Surgical resection for solitary liver metastases may occasionally lead to prolonged survival, especially if the secondary deposit develops years after the primary tumour has been resected.

420 and 421 Colorectal carcinoma. Colonoscopic laser obliteration of obstructing or bleeding tumours of the sigmoid colon or rectum have recently been shown to be a useful palliative procedure in some patients. **420** is a view of a large tumour that has virtually occluded the colonic lumen. **421** was taken after laser treatment, and shows that the colonic lumen has been reopened.

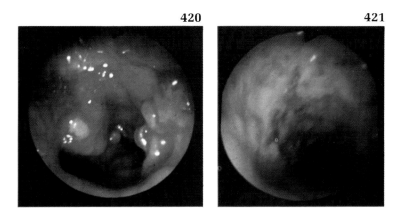

420 **421**

422 Colorectal carcinoma. A recurrence of colorectal carcinoma has occurred at the site of the original resection scar. A small skin metastasis has developed on the right side of the abdomen (left of the photograph).

422

423 Colorectal carcinoma. A photograph of the abdomen of an elderly woman presenting with a huge abdominal mass and fungating tumour within the skin.

423

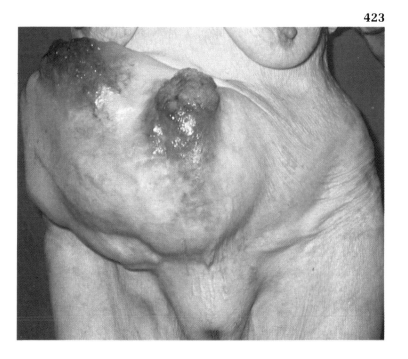

424

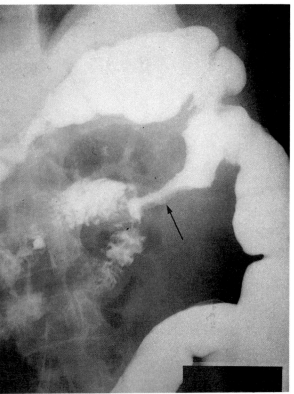

425

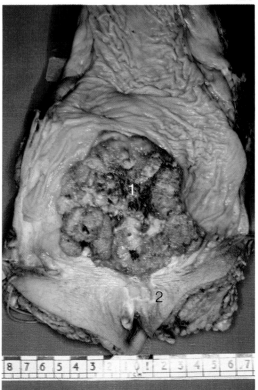

424 Entero-colic fistula shown on barium enema (arrow). A carcinoma of the splenic flexure has formed a fistula with the jejunum, causing profound watery diarrhoea due to bacterial contamination of the small bowel. This type of fistula may only show on barium enema; the track is usually not seen on a barium follow-through.

425 Rectal carcinoma. An abdomino-perineal resection specimen from a patient with an ulcerating polypoid carcinoma of the rectum (1) that had arisen just above the anal margin (2). In this procedure the low sigmoid colon, rectum and anal skin are resected and a permanent colostomy performed. Although abdomino-perineal resection is the only curative procedure for large tumours as close as this to the anal margin, local transrectal excision or electrocoagulation may be indicated for small, mobile tumours.

426

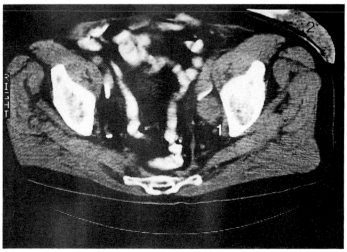

426 Rectal carcinoma. Local pelvic recurrences following abdomino-perineal resection may be difficult to detect clinically. This is a computerised tomographic scan from a patient presenting with pelvic pain 1 year after abdomino-perineal resection for rectal carcinoma. Tumour recurrence is present in the pelvis (1). The colostomy is seen on the left side of the abdominal wall (2).

427 Diverticular disease of the colon. A colonic diverticulum on the left has been opened and emptied of faecal matter. The muscle wall is thickened and pale. Colonic diverticula are usually asymptomatic and are very common in patients over the age of 60 years. They are very rare in parts of the world where dietary fibre intake is high. Diets that are low in fibre result in small stools that require high intracolonic pressures for their propulsion along the colon. The high pressure leads to protrusion of the mucous membrane through vulnerable points in the colonic musculature at the sites where blood vessels penetrate the colonic wall between the mesenteric border and the lateral taeniae coli.

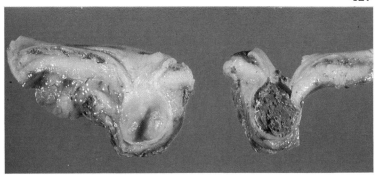

427

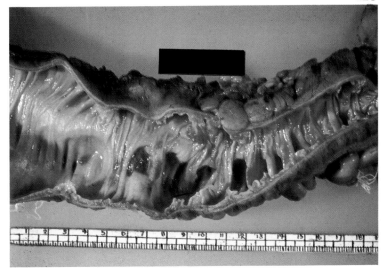

428

428 Diverticular disease of the colon. The descending and sigmoid colon have been opened to show the mucosal surface and the linearly arranged openings of numerous diverticula.

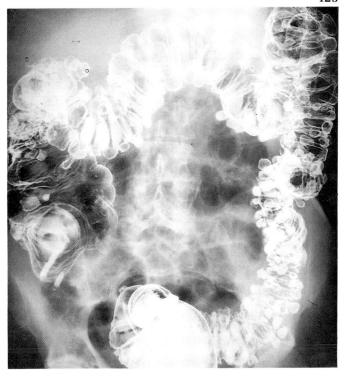

429

429 Diverticular disease of the colon. A barium enema showing multiple large bowel diverticula.

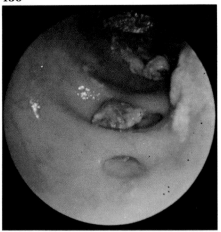

430 Diverticular disease of the colon. A colonoscopic view of diverticulosis of the sigmoid colon. A small faecolith is partially obstructing the neck of one of these diverticula. Diverticulitis is thought to result from obstruction of diverticula by inspissated faecoliths. As the wall of the diverticulum is thin, there is the potential for local peritonitis, with abscess formation. Generalised peritonitis may also develop.

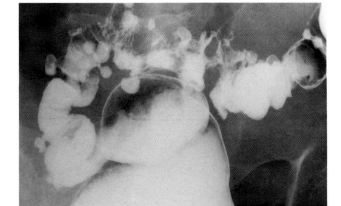

431 Diverticular disease of the colon. A barium enema performed in an elderly woman with recent change in bowel habit. Severe diverticulosis and spasm of the sigmoid colon is seen. It is not possible to exclude a polyp or carcinoma in a patient with an x-ray appearance such as this (see **433**).

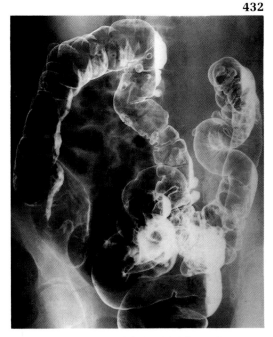

432 Diverticular disease of the colon. A barium enema in a patient presenting with rectal bleeding. Diverticular disease of the colon is present. Rectal haemorrhage is an occasional complication of diverticular disease, but colonic diverticula are common and their presence on barium enema does not necessarily mean that they are the cause of the bleeding. Selective superior and inferior mesenteric arteriography are valuable for investigating patients presenting with an acute rectal bleed. Patients presenting with less severe haemorrhage, or after the bleeding has ceased, should undergo colonoscopy.

433 Diverticular disease of the colon. A colonoscopy has been performed in the same patient as in **431**. A large pedunculated polyp is present in the sigmoid colon, emphasising the need for colonoscopy or flexible sigmoidoscopy in patients thought to have bleeding or change of bowel habit, irrespective of the presence of diverticular disease on barium enema. Colonoscopy should always be performed cautiously in patients with diverticular disease and spasm, as there is the risk of intubating a wide-mouthed diverticulum, causing perforation.

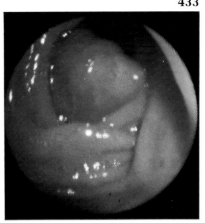

434

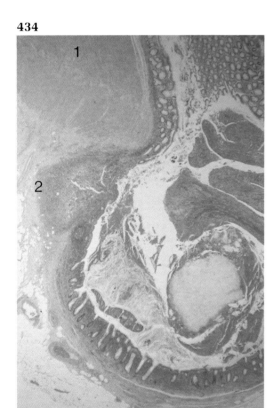

435

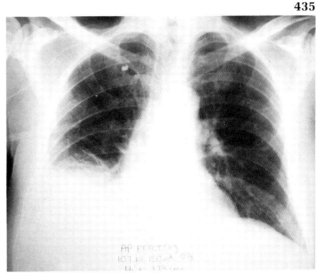

434 Diverticulitis. The lower part of an inflamed colonic diverticulum is shown in this low-power photomicrograph. The colonic muscularis propria is thickened (1) and the mucosa has been lost underneath. The ulcer base (2) consists of inflammatory material in which occasional giant cells (tiny at this magnification) are present. There is a little surrounding fibrosis. The diverticular lumen contains pus and faecal debris.

435 Subphrenic abscess usually results from generalised peritonitis after perforation of abdominal viscera, such as a peptic ulcer, a colonic diverticulum or an inflamed appendix. Patients with subphrenic abscesses may present with a fever of unknown origin or malaise, with loss of appetite and weight, in the absence of localising clinical features. Upper abdominal pain or pleuritic-type chest pain with referral to the shoulder may have been noticed by the patient. This chest x-ray, performed in a patient with a right-sided subphrenic abscess, shows elevation of the right hemi-diaphragm with adjacent collapse of the lung base and a small pleural effusion.

436

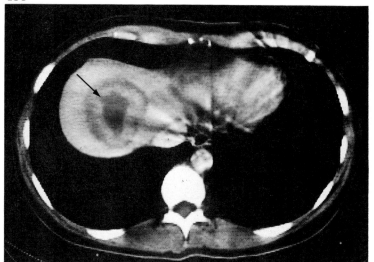

436   Subphrenic abscess.
A computerised tomographic scan
has demonstrated a right-sided
subphrenic abscess (arrow) above
the liver capsule. Ultrasonography
may also be valuable in the
diagnosis of subphrenic abscesses.
Early cases may respond to a short
course of broad-spectrum antibiotic
therapy, but most patients require
percutaneous aspiration or some
form of surgical drainage.

437

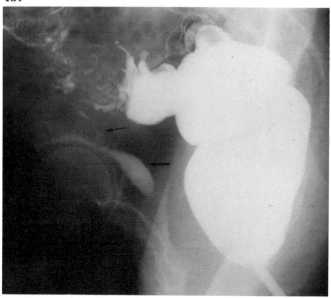

437 and **438   Colo-vesical fistula.**
Fistulae between the sigmoid colon and
bladder are much more common in men
than in women, because of the close
relationship between the two structures.
The most common cause for a
colovesical fistula is diverticular
disease. Less common causes include
Crohn's disease and colorectal
carcinoma. Women suffering from any of
these three disorders may instead
develop a colo-vaginal fistula. **437** is a
barium enema in a man with sigmoid
diverticular disease, illustrating the
small fistulous track between the
sigmoid colon and the bladder vault
(arrows). An erect x-ray performed
during barium enema in another patient
with this complication is shown in **438**.
There is a diagnostic air–contrast fluid
level within the bladder. Patients with
this complication may present with the
passage of air or faeces *per urethra* or
recurrent urinary infections. The
presence of any of these complications
indicates the need for surgical
intervention.

438

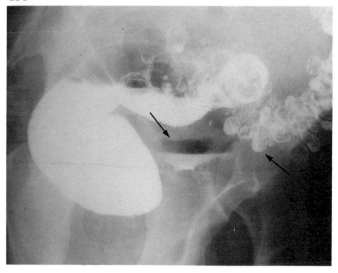

439 'Spastic colon' or irritable bowel syndrome. A particularly bizarre stool, from a young woman with the irritable bowel syndrome, can be seen in the figure. Irritable bowel syndrome is a very common disorder accounting for abdominal symptoms in up to 50% of new referrals to gastroenterology outpatients in the UK. The pathophysiology of this syndrome is poorly understood. The pain has been correlated with colonic spasm and abdominal distension. Alternating constipation and diarrhoea may be associated with abnormalities in small and large bowel transit. Although symptoms from this disorder may be very distressing, there is no structural abnormality of the gastrointestinal tract. It is unusual for symptoms from the syndrome to develop for the first time in patients over the age of 40 years. Symptoms include abdominal pain and distension, which is commonly related to eating or defecation. The pain may be present anywhere in the abdomen. Alternating constipation and diarrhoea is often associated with the frequent passage of stools in the early part of the day. There is wide variation in the character of the stool, which may vary from being partially formed to hard and pellet-like.

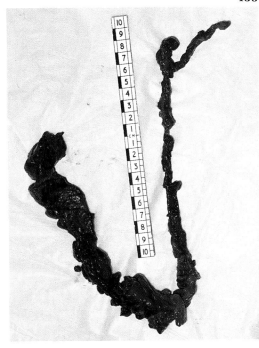

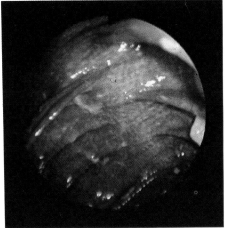

441 Melanosis coli. This colonoscopic view illustrates the black or brown discolouration of the colonic mucosa, which is thought to result from faecal stasis and the use of anthracene laxatives such as senna. The mucosal pigmentation is usually maximal in the rectum and sigmoid colon.

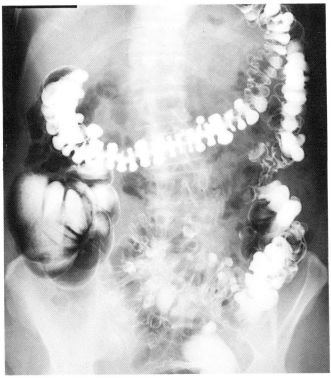

440 Irritable bowel syndrome. The investigation of patients with alteration in bowel habit should include sigmoidoscopy and barium enema. An example of an enema in a patient with irritable bowel syndrome and early diverticular disease is shown here. There are increased haustral markings and spasm, particularly in the transverse colon. A persistent area of spasm may lead the radiologist to be concerned about the possibility of an organic stricture. Intravenous injection of an anticholinergic drug usually relieves the spasm in patients with irritable bowel syndrome undergoing barium enema.

442

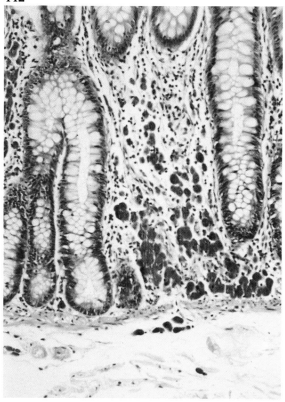

442 to **444** **Melanosis coli.** These sections were taken from a colon that had been resected for carcinoma. This tissue was taken from a place remote from the tumour. The patient had taken laxatives for many years. Many dark macrophages are seen in the lamina propria and in the submucosa just beneath in **442**. The preparation in **443** has been stained with alcian blue–diastase PAS. The macrophages show a red colour because of the lipofuscin-like material within them. **444** shows the results of staining the section with the Masson–Fontana method. This silver-staining technique is usually used to identify melanin, which it colours black. Lipofuscin can also appear black by this method.

443

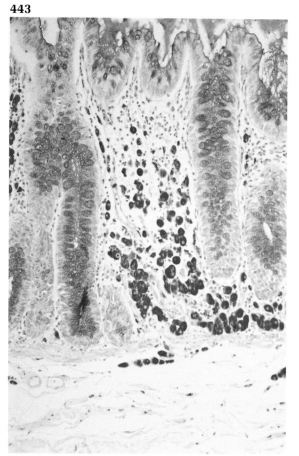

444

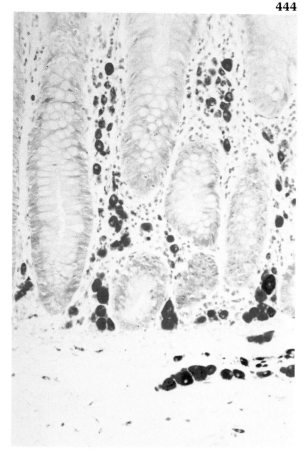

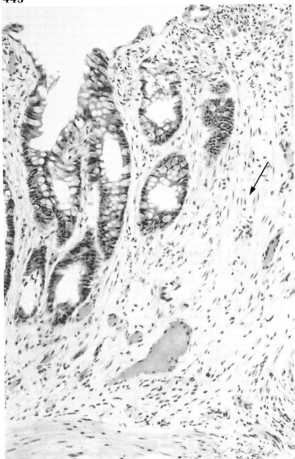

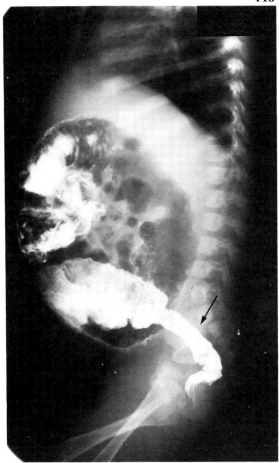

445   Solitary rectal ulcer. A rectal biopsy from a patient who suffered from constipation. This solitary rectal ulcer (a condition in which the lesions may be neither ulcers nor solitary) is considered to be a consequence of straining at stool with prolapse and strangulation of the anterior rectal mucosa. The surface epithelium on the right is eroded and inflamed. The lamina propria is fibrous, and it contains ectatic blood vessels and pale pink strands of spindle-shaped smooth muscle cells which have been drawn upwards (arrow) from the frayed muscularis mucosa below.

446   Hirschsprung's disease. This condition is characterised by the absence of ganglion cells in the bowel wall. Aganglionosis almost always affects the rectum and distal sigmoid colon, but it may extend more proximally. Clinical presentation is usually in the first few days of life with failure to pass meconium and abdominal distension. This is a lateral view of the rectum and colon shown on a barium enema in a six day old infant. The aganglionic segment has been shown clearly (arrow).

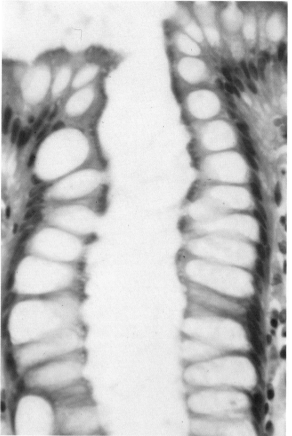

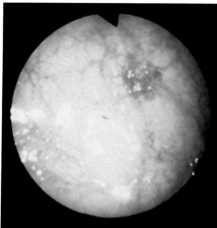

448 Angiodysplasia. These vascular malformations commonly occur in the ascending colon, caecum and terminal ileum of older patients. More-widespread use of angiography and colonoscopy in recent years has demonstrated that these vascular ectasias are a common cause of lower gastrointestinal bleeding in patients over the age of 60 years. This colonoscopic view of the angiodysplastic lesion illustrates a cluster of dilated venules a few millimetres in diameter.

447 Intestinal spirochaetosis. A section of the superficial part of a large intestinal gland seen at high magnification. The surface and upper glandular epithelial luminal border shows a blue (haematoxyphilic) fringe due to the staining peculiarity of the dense coat of intestinal spirochaetes adherent to this area. The clinical significance of these spirochaetes is not known.

449

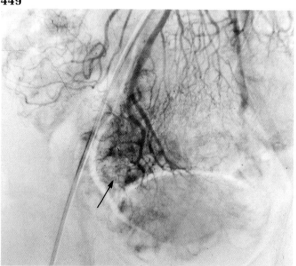

449 Angiodysplasia. Colonoscopy and angiography are the most useful investigations for identifying angiodysplasia. This digital subtraction selective superior mesenteric arteriogram was performed in a patient who had recently suffered from three brisk rectal haemorrhages. Clusters of dilated tortuous angiodysplastic blood vessels are present in the terminal ileum and caecum (arrow). Early venous filling from these arteriovenous communications is another angiographic sign of angiodysplasia. This patient subsequently underwent resection of terminal ileum and caecum. Other approaches to treatment include the application of laser or electrocoagulation directly to the angiodysplastic lesions during colonoscopy.

450   Angiodysplasia. A section of caecal mucosa and submucosa from a patient who underwent a right hemicolectomy for bleeding due to angiodysplasia. The main artery of the specimen was cannulated and filled with barium before the preparation of this section. The barium is seen as the grey material within the dilated, abnormal mucosal and submucosal blood vessels which are characteristic of angiodysplasia.

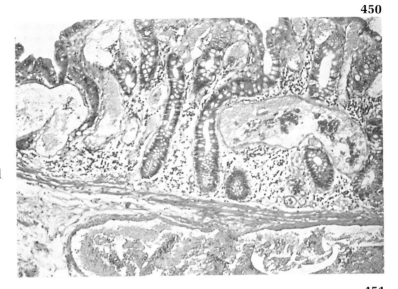

451   Ischaemic colitis is an acute illness presenting with left iliac fossa pain and diarrhoea with dark red rectal bleeding. It is usually seen in patients with a history of generalised arteriosclerosis, or those with a history of risk factors for arterial disease. The colonoscopic appearances are often non-specific. The mucosa may appear dusky blue in colour, with confluent areas of ulceration and oedema. Typically the changes are most marked in the descending colon and splenic flexure.

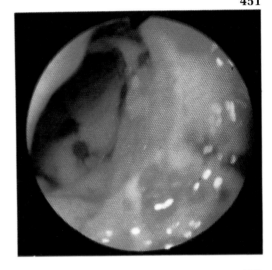

452   Ischaemic colitis. Abnormalities on barium enema will depend on the timing of the investigation in relationship to the duration of symptoms. Small, rounded filling defects are seen in the walls of the descending and sigmoid colon (arrow). This appearance, which may even be visible on plain abdominal radiography, is called 'thumb-printing'.

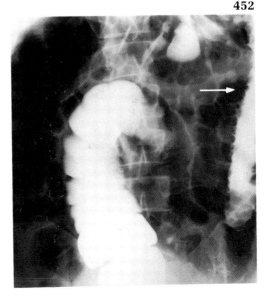

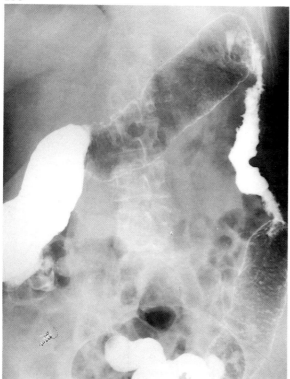

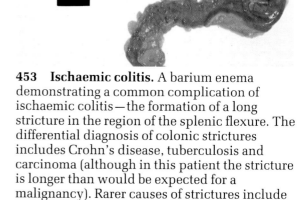

453   Ischaemic colitis. A barium enema demonstrating a common complication of ischaemic colitis—the formation of a long stricture in the region of the splenic flexure. The differential diagnosis of colonic strictures includes Crohn's disease, tuberculosis and carcinoma (although in this patient the stricture is longer than would be expected for a malignancy). Rarer causes of strictures include radiation and amoebiasis.

455

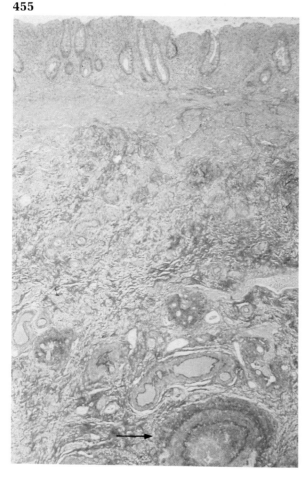

454   Ischaemic colitis. A post-mortem colonic specimen from a patient with ischaemic haemorrhage of the splenic flexure. The patient had died from a myocardial infarction. The usual natural history for ischaemic colitis is one of spontaneous resolution, with healing by fibrosis. Operative resection of the subsequent ischaemic strictures is required only occasionally.

455   Ischaemic colitis. A section of submucosa and mucosa from a patient who underwent resection because of ischaemic disease of the colon. Elastic tissue is stained black and collagen red in this preparation. The epithelium is atrophic, and the submucosa is fibrous. The artery at the bottom of the field (arrow) has been blocked but partial recanalisation has occurred; this is seen as tiny channels within the original lumen of the artery.

456 and **457** **Ischaemic colitis.**
Evidence of haemorrhage into the
mucosa is one of the hallmarks of
ischaemic colitis. When the acute
ischaemia has resolved, evidence
of previous haemorrhage may be
sought by the detection of
haemosiderin-laden macrophages.
456 shows macrophages
containing brown haemosiderin
(arrow). **457** is a higher-
magnification section stained by
Perls' technique: the
haemosiderin deposits appear a
Prussian blue colour because of
their iron content.

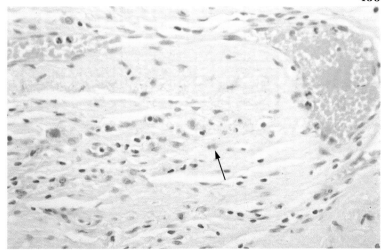

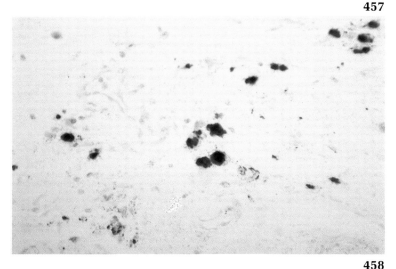

458 **Chronic intestinal ischaemia** is a rare cause of
abdominal pain, weight loss or change of bowel habit.
It is usually seen in patients with a history of arterial
disease elsewhere. The arterial stenoses are usually
seen near the origin of the feeding artery from the
abdominal aorta. This is an oblique view of the
abdominal aorta during digital subtraction angiography
in a patient with chronic upper abdominal pain. There
is a stenosis of the coeliac axis with post-stenotic
dilatation (arrow). Arterial reconstruction may relieve
symptoms, but the results are often disappointing.

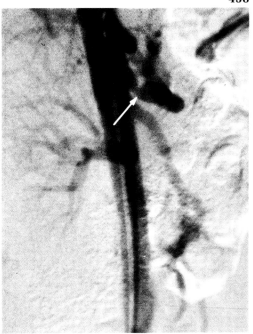

459

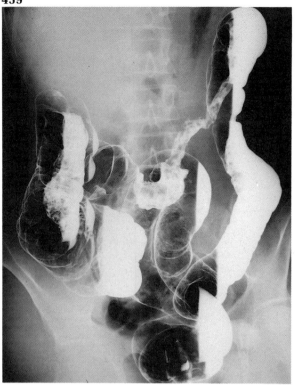

459 and **460** **Radiation damage and the gut.**
A barium enema (**459**) and surgical resection
specimen (**460**) from a patient with a radiation-
induced stricture of the distal transverse colon
2 years after a course of radiotherapy for a
widely infiltrating transitional cell carcinoma of
the left kidney. The stricture had caused
subacute colonic obstruction. The mucosa is
atrophic and there are several large ulcers filled
with haemorrhagic slough and surrounding
oedema. There is distension of the colon
proximal to the stricture. The terminal ileum
and sigmoid colon are liable to irradiation
damage following pelvic malignancy. Modern
radiotherapeutic programmes include
precautions to avoid irradiation enteritis and
colitis. Surgery is indicated for complications
such as intestinal obstruction, fistula formation,
haemorrhage or perforation—but healing is often
poor, with breakdown of anastamoses.

460

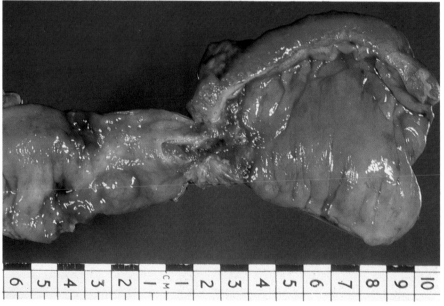

461   Radiation damage of the gut. The wall of small
bowel following irradiation therapy. This preparation
has been stained by the MSB technique. There is
marked submucosal oedema and vascular ectasia due
to irradiation.

461

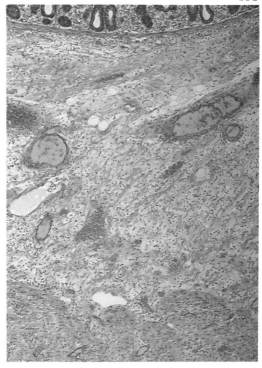

462

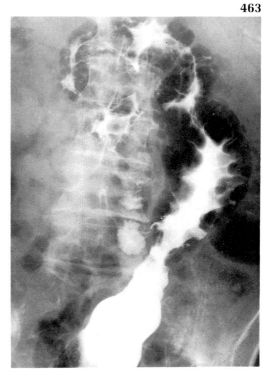

463

462 and **463   Pneumatosis cystoides intestinalis.** This rare disease is characterised by the presence
of gas-filled cysts in the subserosa or submucosa of the colon or ileum. The pathogenesis of the
cysts is unknown, but there is an association with chronic bronchitis and emphysema. The gas-
filled cysts are present in the left colon of this patient with pneumatosis, and may be seen on the
plain abdominal radiograph (**462**). The appearances of the cysts are even more dramatic after
introduction of barium per rectum (**463**). The gas-filled cysts may be several centimetres in
diameter. Patients may present with intestinal obstruction, change of bowel habit or rectal
bleeding. Perforation or significant haemorrhage are rare complications.

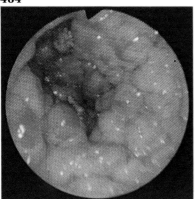

464   Pneumatosis cystoides intestinalis. The displacement of the mucosa by cysts is seen on this colonoscopic view. This condition normally leads a benign course—complications are rare and treatment for asymptomatic patients is unnecessary. Courses of continuous high-flow oxygen therapy may lead to resolution of the cysts, but most patients relapse within 1 year.

465   Pneumatosis cystoides intestinalis. The empty cystic space at the bottom left is lined by giant cells of foreign body type, characteristic of this condition. The mucosa and submucosa nearby show a little chronic inflammation.

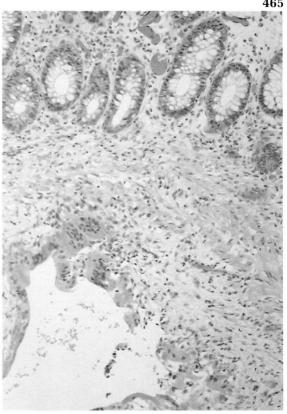

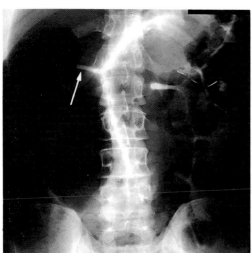

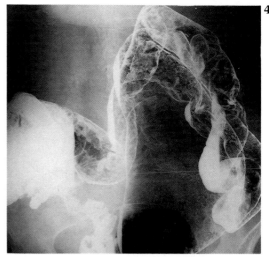

466 and **467   Sigmoid volvulus.** This is a common cause of large bowel obstruction in developing countries, and accounts for about 5% of cases of colonic obstruction in the West. The condition usually develops in patients with an excessively long sigmoid colon and a narrow base to its long mesentery. Subacute episodes of abdominal pain frequently precede the final acute attack. The plain abdominal x-ray (**466**) was obtained from a middle-aged man with a 48h history of colicky abdominal pain and absolute constipation. The markedly dilated sigmoid loop forms the shape of an inverted 'U' and occupies the whole of the central abdominal cavity. The haustral folds appear as thick white lines (arrow). **467** is a barium enema performed in an elderly patient with subacute colonic obstruction due to a sigmoid volvulus. Torsion of the mesenteric vasculature occasionally leads to ischaemic necrosis of the bowel. An uncomplicated sigmoid volvulus may be managed by decompression using a sigmoidoscope or by means of a rubber tube introduced into the volvulus via the sigmoidoscope. Resection of the redundant sigmoid colon is performed when the acute episode has subsided.

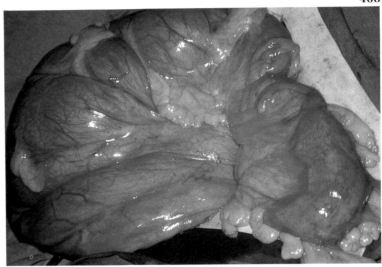

468 **Sigmoid volvulus.** An operative photograph of a sigmoid volvulus, showing the hugely distended sigmoid loop that has become twisted around the neck of its mesentery. This volvulus could not be deflated sigmoidoscopically. Other parts of the colon may be implicated in volvulus formation—a volvulus of the caecum and terminal ileum may develop in patients with an abnormally mobile right colon or congenital malrotation of the bowel.

468

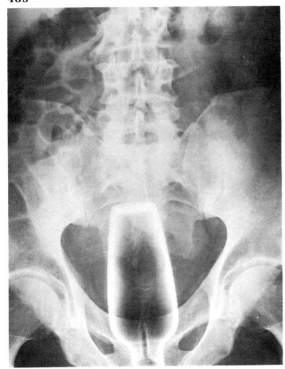

469

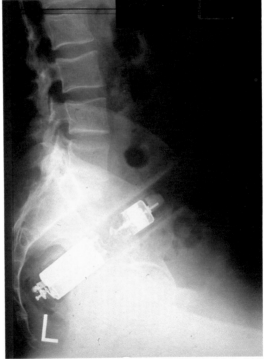

470

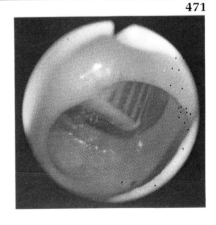

471

469 to **471** **Foreign bodies.** A wide variety of foreign bodies may be encountered in the rectum or sigmoid colon. A plain abdominal x-ray and lateral view should be performed in patients where foreign bodies are suspected. Rectal examination should be performed in the conscious patient. There may be blood on the finger, or the foreign body may be palpated. **469** is a plain pelvic radiograph in a patient with a glass bottle in the rectum. **470** is a lateral pelvic radiograph and **471** a flexible sigmoidoscopic view of a vibrator at the recto-sigmoid junction. Haemorrhage or perforation may result from the insertion of foreign bodies and from attempts at their removal.

472

473

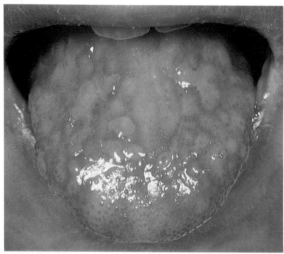
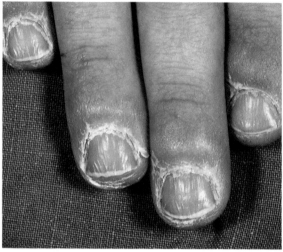

472 and **473**   **Graft-versus-host disease (GVHD).** This complication of bone marrow transplantation is believed to be mediated by cytotoxic T-lymphocytes of donor origin. Acute GVHD is seen in the first 2 months after transplantation. Diarrhoea, with ulceration of the mouth and tongue (**472**) and exfoliative dermatitis (**473**) may accompany the more severe forms of the disease. In patients with diarrhoea, sigmoidoscopy may show friable mucosa with contact bleeding and, occasionally, ulceration. Rectal biopsy is helpful in the differential diagnosis, but must be avoided in patients with a low platelet count or a prolonged bleeding time. Treatment with high doses of intravenous methylprednisolone may control the disease, but established acute GVHD carries a high mortality.

474

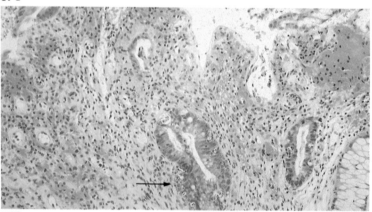

475

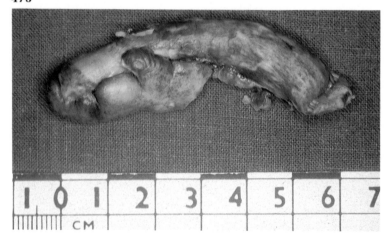

474   Graft-versus-host disease. A rectal biopsy section from a patient who suffered GVHD in the course of bone marrow transplantation for leukaemia. The mucosa is inflamed and eroded. Some glands show lymphocytic permeation and marked degeneration of scattered epithelial cells near to the permeating lymphocytes (arrow). This type of epithelial destruction characterises GVHD in general, as well as in this site.

475   Acute appendicitis. A resected appendix from a patient with acute appendicitis.

476   Acute appendicitis. The lumen of this appendix contains pus (arrow). The mucosa is haemorrhagic and ulcerated. A sprinkling of acute inflammatory cells is seen throughout the rest of the appendiceal wall.

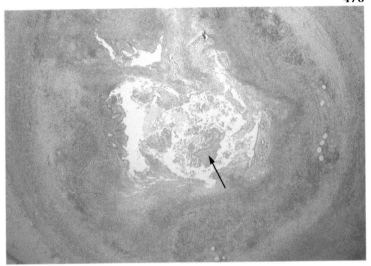

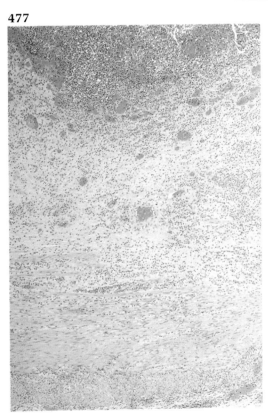

477   Acute appendicitis. In this section there is transmural acute inflammation from the haemorrhagic mucosa above to the muscular coat of the organ below.

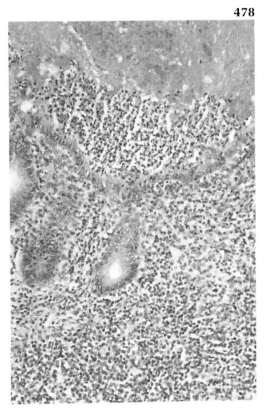

478   Acute appendicitis, showing the early mucosal inflammation that precedes the occurrence of advanced mucosal destruction seen in **477**. A purulent exudate and faecal material are seen at the top, and preliminary stages of active mucosal inflammation are seen in the centre.

479

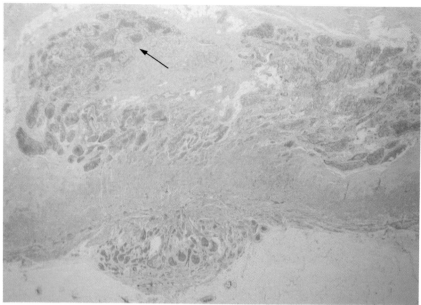

479 Appendiceal carcinoid tumours. These are commonly found in appendicectomy specimens. In this section the lumen of the appendix has been obliterated and islands of tumour are seen in the remaining fibrofatty tissue (arrow). Tumour has permeated the muscular wall of the appendix and there is early infiltration of mesoappendix below.

480

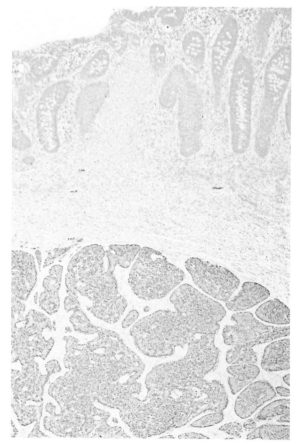

480 Appendiceal carcinoid tumours. This section of carcinoid tumour and intact overlying mucosa has been stained for silver using the Linder method. The nests of tumour cells are darkly stained in the lower half of the field. The argyrophilia of appendiceal carcinoid tumours is a reflection of their endocrine nature.

CHAPTER 12

Inflammatory Bowel Disease

481

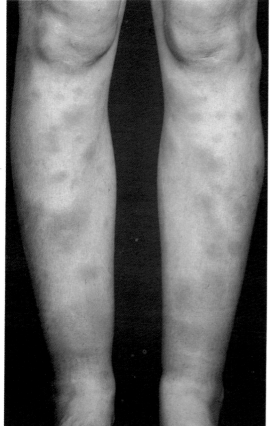

482

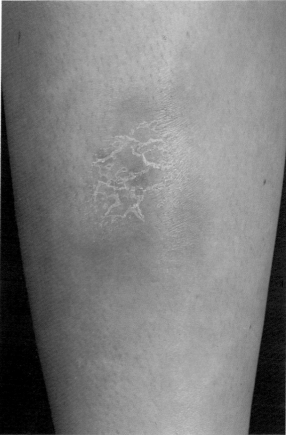

481 and **482** **Erythema nodosum.** This inflammation of small blood vessels in the deep dermis and subcutaneous tissue gives rise to characteristic tender red swellings on the front of the shins, and occasionally on the thighs and forearms. It can occur in association with ulcerative colitis and Crohn's disease, as well as *Streptococcal* infection, leprosy, tuberculosis, sarcoidosis and drugs. The lesions usually last for 2–4 weeks, although they have a tendency to recur in some patients. The more chronic lesions may develop a violaceous appearance, or any of the colours of a resolving bruise. Corticosteroid treatment reduces the swelling and fever but does not hasten the clearing of the lesion.

483

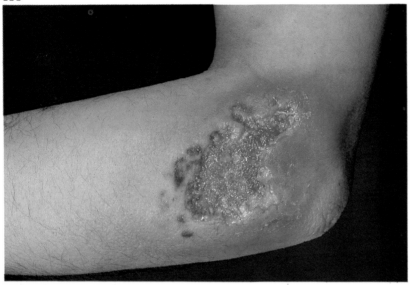

484

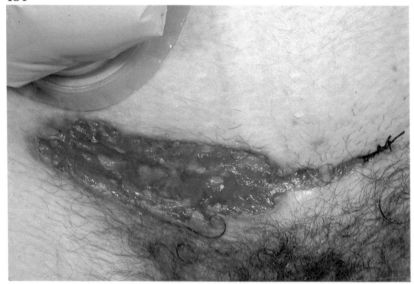

483 and **484** **Pyoderma gangrenosum.** In this condition necrotic
ulcers with characteristic violaceous edges may extend rapidly,
destroying large areas of the skin. The ulceration has a tendency to
occur within scars. **484** illustrates this phenomenon in the Caesarian
section scar of a patient with Crohn's disease and an ileostomy (the
sutures on the right follow a diagnostic biopsy (**485** and **486**).
Although ulcerative colitis and Crohn's disease are the most
common associations with pyoderma gangrenosum, rheumatoid
arthritis, multiple myeloma and Wegener's granulomatosis may also
be complicated by pyoderma. Occasionally there is an underlying
infective aetiology, such as amoebiasis, tuberculosis or nocardiosis.
Successful treatment of pyoderma gangrenosum depends on
controlling the underlying disease. Any suspicion of an infective
causation such as amoebiasis requires the appropriate investigations
and treatment. High-dose corticosteroids should be instituted in
patients with ulcerative colitis or Crohn's disease and pyoderma
gangrenosum. Colectomy usually leads to a remission of pyoderma
in patients with ulcerative colitis or Crohn's disease.

485 and **486** **Pyoderma gangrenosum.** A section from the skin of a patient with pyoderma in association with inflammatory bowel disease. There is an ulcer on the left of **485**; its base is composed of chronic inflammatory cells and fibrous tissue. The two small blood vessels in the ulcer base (bottom centre of **485**) can be seen at higher power in **486**. The vessel on the left is intact, but that on the right is being destroyed by a vasculitic process.

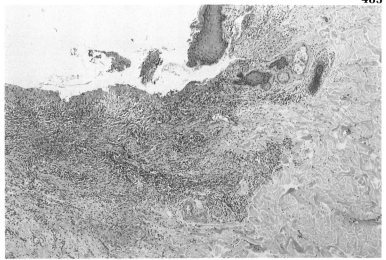

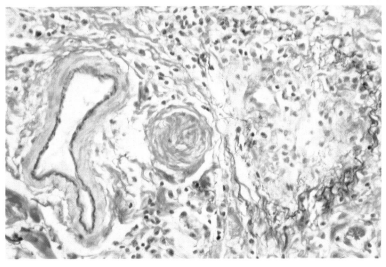

487 **Episcleritis.** Painful inflammation of the optic sclera may be associated with inflammatory bowel disease. Severe inflammation may be accompanied by keratitis, photophobia or uveitis.

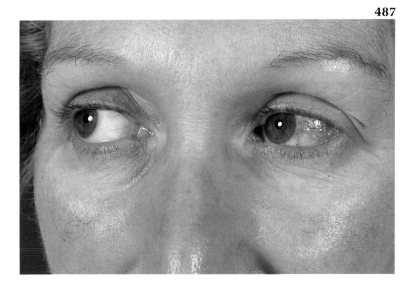

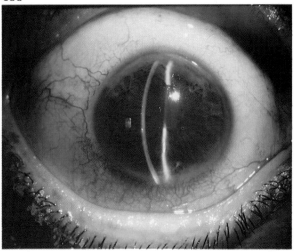

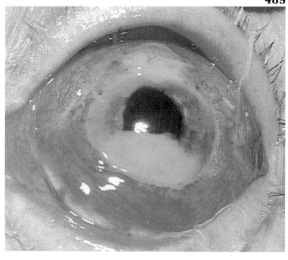

488   Uveitis. This figure illustrates acute anterior uveitis. Patients usually present with a history of a few days of redness, pain and photophobia in one eye. Conjunctival hyperaemia has spread to the edges of the cornea.

489   Uveitis. Very severe attacks of acute anterior uveitis may produce a fibrin clot with inflammatory debris in the anterior chamber. This is known as a hypopyon. In the figure inflammatory debris has accumulated within the anterior chamber, giving rise to a hypopyon with its characteristic fluid level. Severe complicated forms of anterior uveitis occur rarely in patients with inflammatory bowel disease.

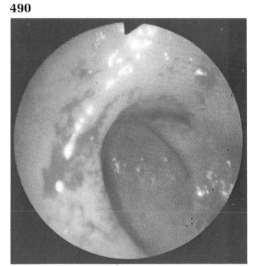

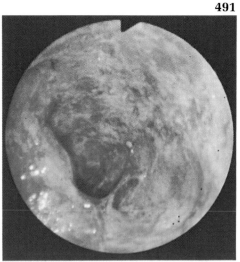

490   Ulcerative colitis. This colonoscopic view in a patient with mild ulcerative colitis illustrates the mucosal oedema and a loss of the normal colonic vascular pattern (compare with normal colonic appearances in Chapter 10). This photograph was taken on withdrawal of a colonoscope from the region. Contact between the colonoscope and the mucosa has given rise to contact bleeding.

491   Ulcerative colitis. More severe changes of ulcerative colitis are seen on this colonoscopic view. Many small confluent ulcers with overlying slough and mucus are seen. Colonoscopy was performed in this patient several weeks after clinical recovery. Colonoscopy in patients with severely active ulcerative colitis is associated with an increased risk of perforation.

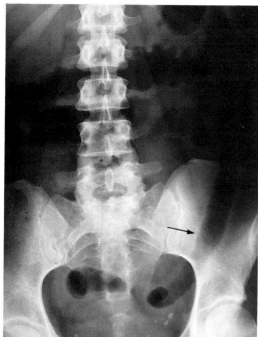

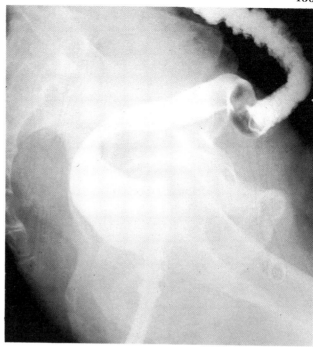

492   Ulcerative colitis. Plain abdominal x-rays are valuable in the assessment of patients with severely active ulcerative colitis. In this patient a shortened tubular colon with loss of haustra is seen (arrow). It must be emphasised that this is a plain film of unprepared bowel—it is an ominous appearance suggesting active colitis throughout the empty colon (see **509** for more-severe 'toxic dilatation of the colon').

493   Ulcerative colitis. A lateral view of the pelvis in a patient with ulcerative colitis undergoing barium enema. The presacral space (between the barium-filled rectum and the sacrum) is widened.

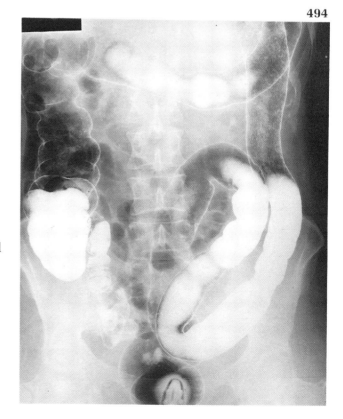

494   Ulcerative colitis. A barium enema showing a tubular colon with loss of haustral pattern. The disease extends as far as the proximal transverse colon. The rest of the colon appears spared. Barium has refluxed into the terminal ileum. Ulcerative colitis almost invariably involves the rectum, and extends proximally. Patients in whom the barium enema suggests extensive involvement (as far as the hepatic flexure) run an increased risk of colonic carcinoma ten years or more after diagnosis.

495

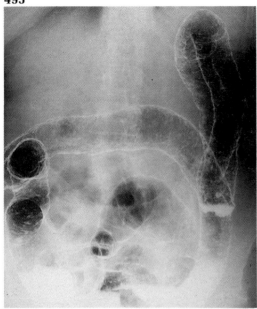

495 Ulcerative colitis. A barium enema showing severe ulcerative colitis, with large ulcers extending throughout the colon. The early changes are those of a fine granular ulceration. Later the mucosa becomes nodular with confluent ulceration. The colonic lumen becomes narrow and its walls become less distensible.

496

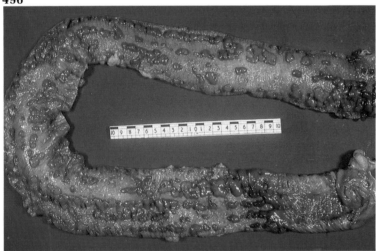

496 Ulcerative colitis. This is a colonic resection specimen from a patient with severe ulcerative colitis that failed to settle on medical treatment. Most of the colonic mucosa has been lost as a result of the inflammatory process, leaving only small islands of visible oedematous mucosa. Sometimes these mucosal islands are visible on a plain abdominal x-ray—their presence suggests a severe colitis.

497

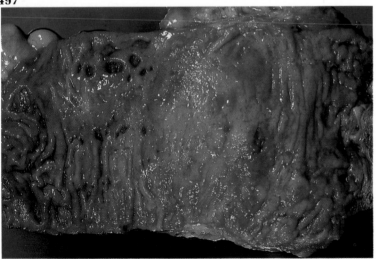

497 Ulcerative colitis. Another resection specimen from a patient with severe ulcerative colitis. Most of the mucosa has been preserved, but punched-out ulcers are seen. Ulcers such as these may penetrate the muscle and serosa, resulting in colonic perforation. An important part of the management of severe fulminant ulcerative colitis is to be able to assess when colectomy is necessary in order to prevent perforation.

498 **Ulcerative colitis.** Section of a colectomy specimen from a patient with fulminant ulcerative colitis. The mucosa shows active inflammation with the formation of a crypt abscess (arrow). The glands show architectural disturbance, and there is congestion of the lamina propria. In this fulminant colitis there is also inflammation and oedema in the submucosa.

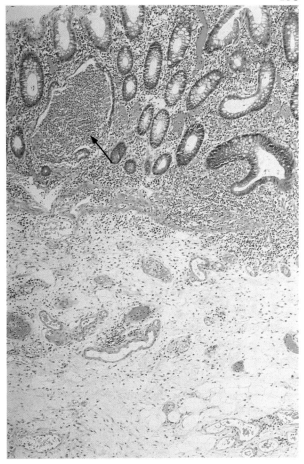

499

499 **Chronic ulcerative colitis.** Inflammation is limited to the mucosa in this patient with chronic ulcerative colitis. Active, acute inflammation is not evident in this rectal biopsy. The muscularis mucosa shows reactive thickening. Several lymphoid aggregates separate the gland bases from the muscularis mucosa, indicating mucosal glandular atrophy. The glands have a jumbled, disorganised appearance.

500

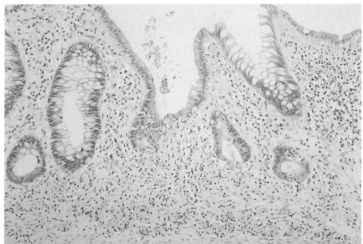

500 Inactive ulcerative colitis.
This rectal biopsy section demonstrates the features of epithelial atrophy. The glands are widely separated from each other and from the muscularis mucosa below. The glandular architecture is irregular. Neither active nor chronic inflammation are seen.

501

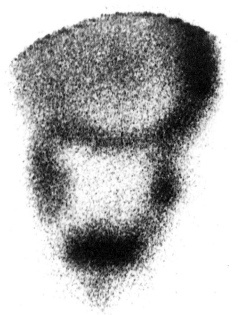

502

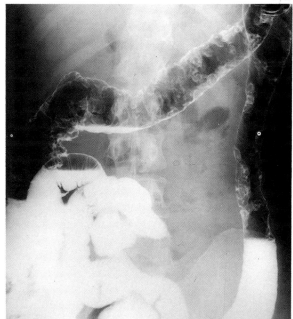

501 Ulcerative colitis. An ^{111}In granulocyte scan of the anterior abdomen in an active total colitis, showing extensive abnormal activity in the whole of the large bowel in addition to normal uptake in the spleen (top right) and liver (top left). The technique is performed by labelling the patient's own leucocytes with ^{111}In, re-injecting them into the patient and performing serial scans over several hours. Although the technique is time-consuming and technically complex, it is non-invasive and particularly suitable for assessing the extent and degree of inflammation in acutely ill patients. It may also be useful in detecting small perforations or abscesses.

502 Ulcerative colitis. A barium enema in a patient with total colitis, demonstrating mucosal irregularity due to pseudopolyp formation. Pseudopolyps and small inflammatory polyps may form from heaped-up areas of granulation tissue.

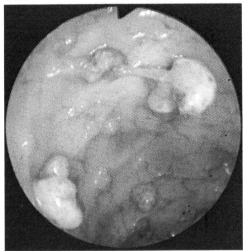

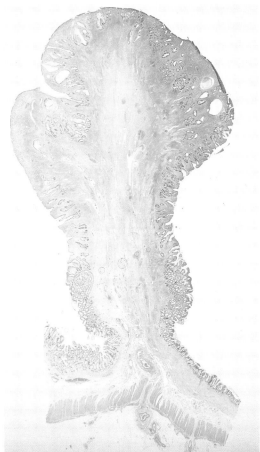

503 Ulcerative colitis: pseudopolyps.
A colonoscopic view of multiple pseudopolyps in a patient with chronic inactive ulcerative colitis. Note that the vascular pattern between the pseudopolyps is only slightly abnormal, and there is no mucosal oedema.

504 Ulcerative colitis: pseudopolyps. A section from a resection specimen of a patient who underwent proctocolectomy for ulcerative colitis. A large inflammatory polyp is seen. It consists of a connective tissue core covered by inflamed, regenerative large bowel mucosa, which in places appears hyperplastic.

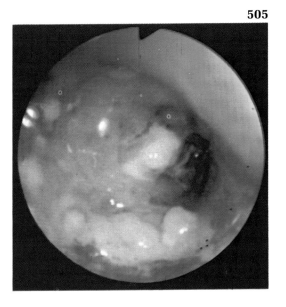

505 Ulcerative colitis and colonic carcinoma. This colonoscopy was performed in a patient with a 30-year history of extensive ulcerative colitis and known mucosal dysplasia (see **508**). She had declined a colectomy 4 years previously.
A carcinoma has developed in the hepatic flexure, almost obstructing the colonic lumen. The risk of carcinoma is greatest in patients with colitis extending to the hepatic flexure or more proximally. The risk of carcinoma increases with increasing duration of the disease, and is of the order of 15% after 30 years in patients with extensive colitis.

506

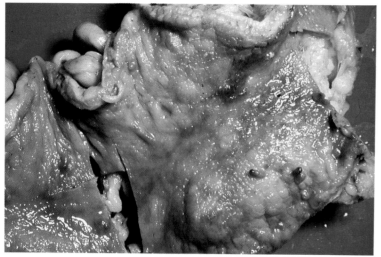

506 Ulcerative colitis and colonic carcinoma. A post-mortem photograph of a colon from a patient with ulcerative colitis and carcinoma. The figure illustrates the potential difficulty in diagnosing a carcinoma in a patient with ulcerative colitis. The carcinoma is flat and plaque-like. There is no ulcerating or polypoid lesion protruding into the lumen.

507

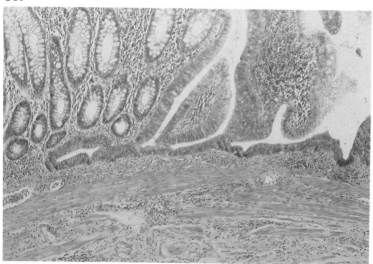

507 and 508 Ulcerative colitis. 507 is a section from a colon in a patient with ulcerative colitis. The mucosa on the left of the picture shows the typical features of an inactive colitis. The mucosa on the right of the photograph has undergone severe epithelial dysplasia. This histological change is thought to be associated with a considerable likelihood of a carcinoma elsewhere in the colon. It is considered that the carcinoma (1) arises from epithelial dysplasia (2), as illustrated in 508. The assessment of mild epithelial dysplasia is highly subjective, and may be difficult in the presence of active inflammation from the colitis. For this reason surveillance colonoscopy with multiple mucosal biopsy specimens is best performed when the disease is in an inactive phase. There is still considerable controversy regarding the frequency with which patients with extensive long-standing ulcerative colitis should undergo colonoscopy. There is an argument for prophylactic colectomy in young patients with long-standing extensive colitis who are at very high risk of developing a carcinoma in middle age.

508

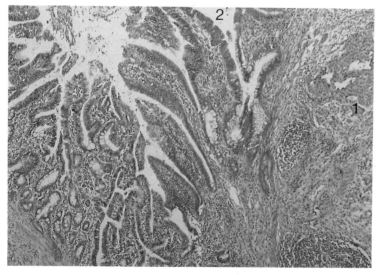

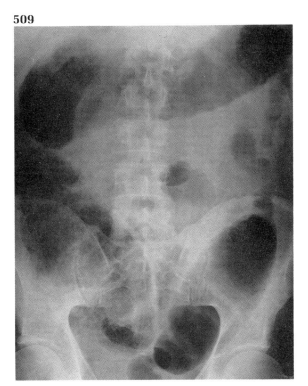

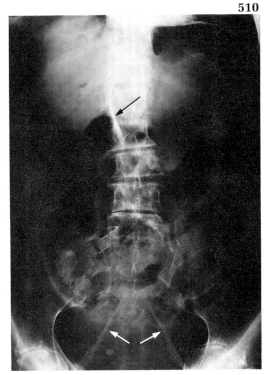

509 Toxic megacolon. A plain abdominal radiograph is necessary in every patient with acute severe symptoms from colitis, because toxic megacolon may be present. The finding of a dilated colon (greater than 5.5 cm in diameter) in an ill patient with tachycardia, pyrexia, abdominal tenderness and diminished bowel sounds confirms the presence of a toxic megacolon. Daily plain abdominal x-ray should be performed in such patients while they receive intensive intravenous treatment with prednisolone, fluid and electrolyte replacement and/or parenteral nutrition.

510 Perforated toxic megacolon. A plain abdominal x-ray in a patient with ulcerative colitis and a perforated toxic megacolon. Free intraperitoneal gas has accumulated under both diaphragms and has outlined the falciform and umbilical ligaments (arrows).

511 Primary sclerosing cholangitis. This condition is characterised by multiple strictures and bead-like dilatations of the intrahepatic and extrahepatic biliary tree. About 70% of patients with primary sclerosing cholangitis are found to have ulcerative colitis, but only about 1% of patients with ulcerative colitis have cholangitis. Endoscopic retrograde cholangiography is the most helpful diagnostic test, as in this patient. The condition usually presents with cholangitis or painless cholestatic jaundice. Some patients may have no symptoms. Bile duct adenocarcinoma is a late complication.

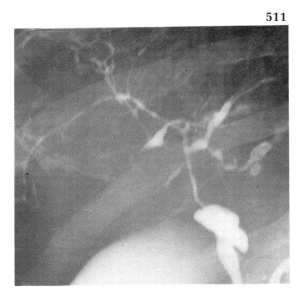

512

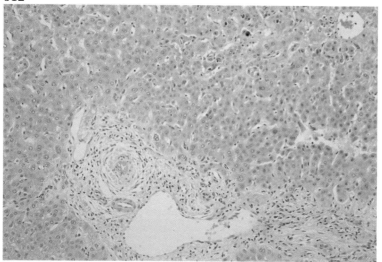

512   Primary sclerosing cholangitis. A section of liver from a patient with sclerosing cholangitis in association with inflammatory bowel disease. There is a centrilobular vein in the upper right corner of the field, with bile plugs towards the centre indicating cholestasis. At the bottom centre of the field there is a portal tract and a large space representing the portal venule. Immediately to the left of the venule is the hepatic arteriole and just above this is the bile ductule which shows the 'onion skin' concentric fibrosis characteristic of sclerosing cholangitis.

513

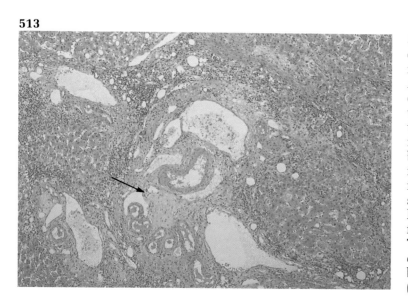

513 and 514   Primary sclerosing cholangitis. These sections show more advanced disease than **512**. A hepatic arteriole lies in the centre of **513**, with a portal venule to the right. Underneath and to the left is a pale pink round scar indicating the site of a destroyed bile ductule (arrow). Chronic inflammatory cells have infiltrated the portal tract, and its surrounding parenchyma. **514** is a higher-power view of the same field with collagen stained red. The scarred remains of the bile ductule (arrows) can be seen below the hepatic arteriole (arrow).

514

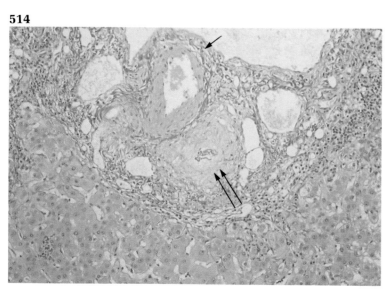

515 **Sacroiliitis.** Ankylosing spondylitis (arrows), or isolated sacroiliitis, are sometimes associated with ulcerative colitis. Patients who suffer from both ulcerative colitis and ankylosing spondylitis usually have the human leucocyte antigen HLA-B27. Sometimes asymptomatic sacroiliitis is discovered at the time of a barium enema or urogram (**543**).

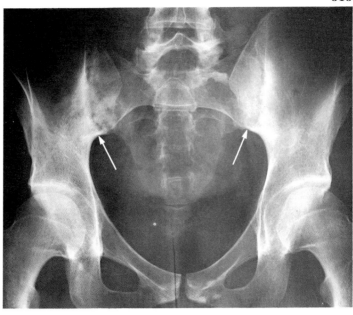

516 **Sulphasalazine sensitivity.** Sulphasalazine is sulphapyridine covalently bound to 5-aminosalicylic acid. It is of value both in the treatment of attacks of ulcerative colitis and in preventing disease relapse. Approximately 10% of patients with ulcerative colitis fail to tolerate sulphasalazine, usually because of the development of a rash, as in this case. The rashes, which are usually attributable to the sulphonamide, vary in morphology from localised itchy maculopapular eruptions to erythema multiforme and the Stevens–Johnson syndrome. This patient suffered generalised erythema multiforme that resolved on stopping sulphasalazine. New drugs such as mesalazine and olsalazine contain only the aspirin-like moiety. These drugs are usually well tolerated by sulphasalazine sensitive patients, provided that they are not sensitive to aspirin.

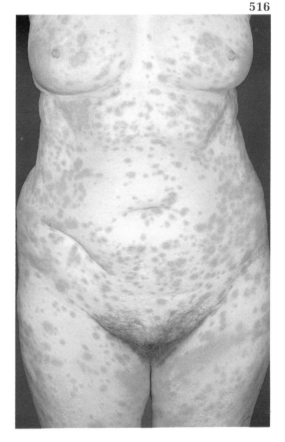

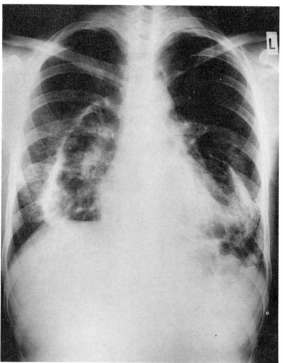 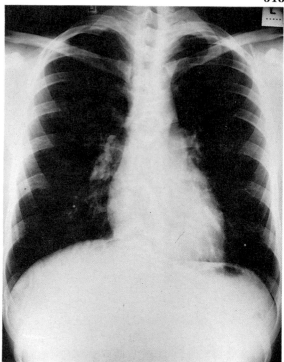

517 and **518**   **Sulphasalazine sensitivity. 517** is a chest x-ray from a patient who developed alveolitis due to sulphasalazine. The changes resolved within 1 week of stopping the drug (**518**). Other unwanted side-effects of sulphasalazine include hypersensitivity rashes, fever, haemolytic anaemia and reversible male infertility due to oligospermia.

519

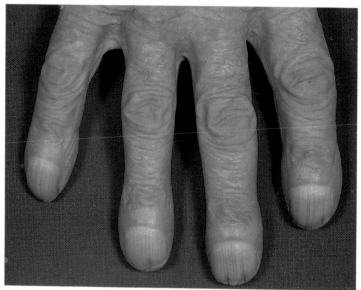

519   **Finger clubbing** is usually idiopathic, but it may indicate chronic cardiac or respiratory disease. Abdominal associations include chronic liver disease and disease of the small intestine—especially coeliac disease or Crohn's disease.

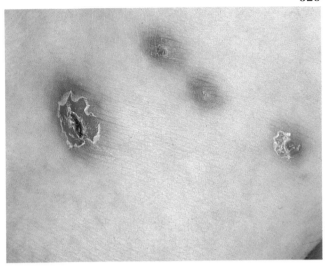

520 Crohn's disease. Crohn's disease is a chronic relapsing inflammatory condition that may occur anywhere in the gastrointestinal tract. Dermatological complications include erythema nodosum and pyoderma gangrenosum. Very rarely skin lesions develop which contain non-caseating granulomas on histology and are therefore more akin to the histological lesion of Crohn's disease found in the bowel. This patient was thought to have pyoderma gangrenosum, although no evidence of Crohn's disease was found on investigation. Biopsy of the lesions showed non-caseating granulomata. Three years later he developed ileo-colonic Crohn's disease.

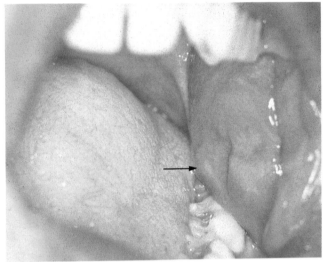

521 Crohn's disease. A photograph of the oral mucosa of a patient with colonic Crohn's disease. There is thickening and fissuring of the mucosa, with a linear fissuring ulcer (arrow). Treatment of the oral lesions includes topical and systemic corticosteroids.

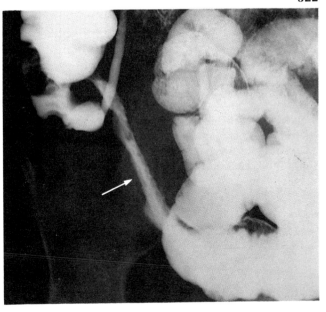

522 Crohn's disease. A small bowel meal demonstrating a long stricture of the terminal ileum (arrow). The differential diagnosis of this appearance includes Crohn's disease, tuberculosis and lymphoma. Laparoscopy or laparotomy may be required for diagnosis, especially in non-Caucasian patients. About 30% of patients with Crohn's disease have exclusively small bowel involvement, 30% have colonic involvement alone, and 40% have combined small and large bowel disease.

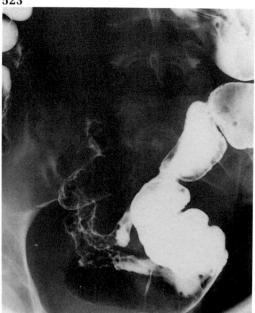

523 Crohn's disease. This small bowel meal has shown several loops of narrowed and ulcerated terminal ileum lying within the right iliac fossa. This phenomenon commonly leads to an inflammatory mass that may be palpable on physical examination.

524

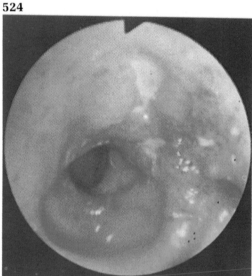

524 Crohn's disease. A colonoscope has been passed through the ileo-caecal valve into the terminal ileum. The mucosa of the terminal ileum is oedematous and inflamed, and a large longitudinal ulcer is visible superiorly. Interestingly, this patient had not had any symptoms for more than 5 years.

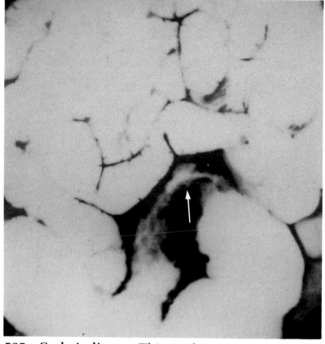

525 Crohn's disease. This single-contrast study illustrates the problems that may arise in the interpretation of mucosal abnormalities in loops of small intestine. However, the study did demonstrate a localised ileal stricture with the characteristic cobblestoning of the mucosa and a few deep 'rosethorn' ulcers (arrow), with surrounding lack of contrast due to thickening of the bowel wall.

526 Crohn's disease. A small bowel meal in a patient with Crohn's disease who had required two previous small intestinal resections. The study was performed because she had suffered several episodes of colicky abdominal pain and vomiting, which had suggested small intestinal obstruction. The investigation demonstrated four strictures of the terminal ileum in the centre of this radiograph with dilated but otherwise normal loops of bowel between them. The term 'skip lesions' is given to areas of involvement with Crohn's disease between areas of normal intestine. Skip lesions strongly suggest the diagnosis of Crohn's disease. Small intestinal obstruction should be treated conservatively in the first instance. Surgery for obstruction due to stricture formation should be considered once the acute episode has settled. Some patients with surprisingly narrow strictures can be maintained on a low-residue diet for many years without surgical intervention.

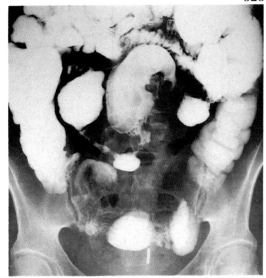

527 C-reactive protein. When patients with Crohn's disease are followed-up in clinics, their physician will normally order blood tests to determine the activity of the intestinal inflammation. The erythrocyte sedimentation rate rises when intestinal inflammation is active, because there is an acute-phase response. Most patients with active Crohn's disease secrete certain proteins into the serum as part of the non-specific acute-phase response to chronic inflammation. The figure shows the results of rocket gel-electrophoresis measurement of serum C-reactive protein in patients with Crohn's disease. The long 'rockets' represent patients with active disease (the bottom four samples on the right are standards).

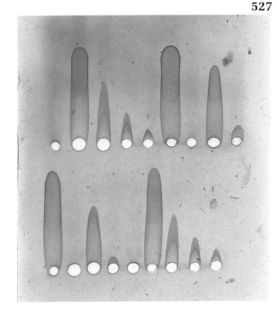

528 Crohn's disease. A surgical resection specimen from a young woman with Crohn's disease and subacute intestinal obstruction. The terminal ileum (on the right of the photograph) joins the caecum on the left. The terminal ileum is grossly thickened and inflamed (arrow), and the mucosa has a cobblestone appearance except in the few centimetres proximal to the ileo-caecal valve.

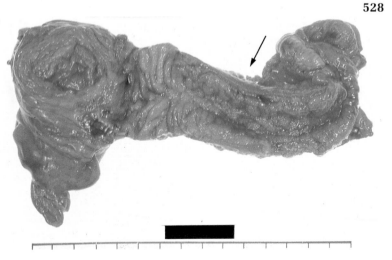

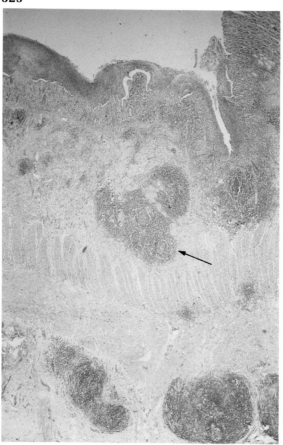

529 Crohn's disease of terminal ileum. The bowel wall is thickened and there is transmural chronic inflammation with darkly staining lymphoid aggregates. Three small granulomas appear lightly stained within the lymphoid aggregate in the centre of the picture (arrow). There is fibrous thickening of the submucosa and serosa around these areas of chronic inflammation. The mucosa is inflamed and ulcerated, and there is an early fissure on the right.

530

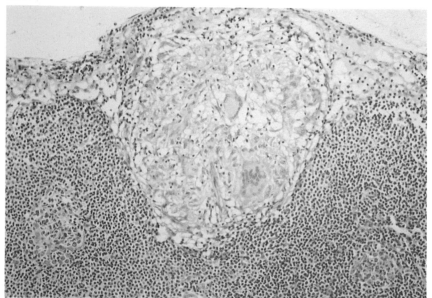

530 Crohn's disease. Part of a mesenteric lymph node taken from a resection of ileum from a patient with Crohn's disease. A well-formed granuloma including occasional giant cells is seen in the subcapsular cortex. Granulomas are commonly seen in lymph nodes draining areas of bowel affected by Crohn's disease. However, other causes of granulomatous inflammation such as tuberculosis should be excluded before making a histological diagnosis of Crohn's disease.

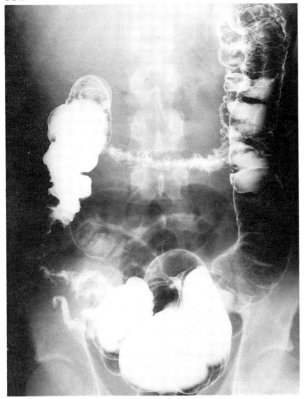

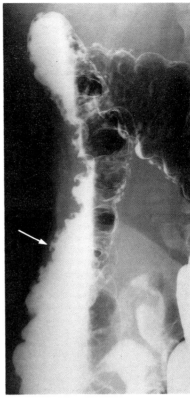

531 Crohn's colitis. A barium enema performed in a young man presenting with colicky abdominal pain and bloody diarrhoea. Rigid sigmoidoscopy and rectal biopsy had been normal and stool cultures were negative. The caecum and transverse colon are narrowed and ulcerated. The distal ascending colon and hepatic flexure are normal. The deep ulceration and normal mucosa between the two skip lesions are virtually diagnostic of Crohn's disease.

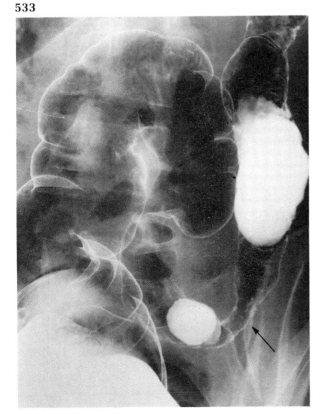

532 Crohn's colitis. A higher-magnification view of the mucosal detail demonstrated on a barium enema in a patient with Crohn's disease of the ascending and transverse colon. Again an irregular mucosal pattern and deep 'collar-stud' ulcers have been demonstrated (arrow).

533 Crohn's colitis. This barium enema has shown a 4 cm stricture at the junction of the descending and sigmoid colon (arrow).

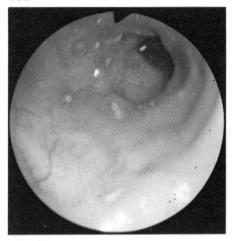

534 **Crohn's colitis.** A colonoscopic view of the descending colon in a patient with Crohn's colitis. There are small ulcers with surrounding erythema, but the vascular pattern of the adjacent mucosa is preserved. Discrete ulcers of this kind are referred to as aphthoid ulcers, akin to the oral aphthous ulcers that occur in some patients with Crohn's disease. This mucosal appearance contrasts with the confluent reddening and oedema that is seen in ulcerative colitis (see **491**).

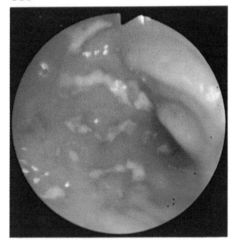

535 **Crohn's colitis.** This colonoscopic photograph was taken in the ascending colon from the same patient as **534**. There is severe disease, as evidenced by large longitudinal ulcers. The main role of colonoscopy in patients with Crohn's disease is in making the original diagnosis and obtaining material for histological confirmation. Although patients with Crohn's disease run an increased risk of adenocarcinoma of the colon, the risk is not nearly as great as that for patients with ulcerative colitis, and is not sufficiently large to warrant regular colonoscopic surveillance of patients with long-standing Crohn's disease.

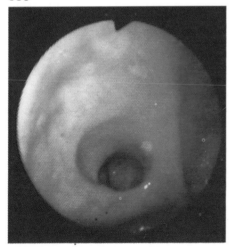

536 **Crohn's disease.** This colonoscopic photograph was obtained in a patient who had undergone resection of the caecum and terminal ileum with an end-to-end ileo-colonic anastomosis. There is a stricture at the anastomosis, with surrounding aphthoid ulcers. It is now recognised that colonoscopy can detect recurrence at the site of intestinal anastomosis in most patients with Crohn's disease soon after resection, although it is often many years before symptoms recur. The cumulative probability of re-operation is about 80% at 20 years after first and second resections. Nowadays surgery is usually reserved for the treatment of complications (fistulae, obstruction due to stricture, and the rarer complications of free perforation and haemorrhage).

537 and **538** **Crohn's disease.** The plain abdominal
x-ray in **537** and the computerised tomographic scan
in **538** were obtained from a patient with Crohn's
colitis, fever and rapidly enlarging mass in the left
side of the abdomen. The plain abdominal x-ray is
valuable in patients where subacute obstruction or
toxic megacolon are suspected. In this patient the
transverse colon is dilated proximal to a narrowed
descending colon (arrow). In **538** the computerised
tomographic scan shows that the thickened
descending colon is surrounded by an abscess cavity
(arrow). Localised perforation and abscess formation
may complicate Crohn's disease, and the symptoms
may be masked by corticosteroid treatment.

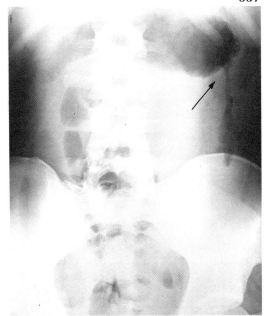

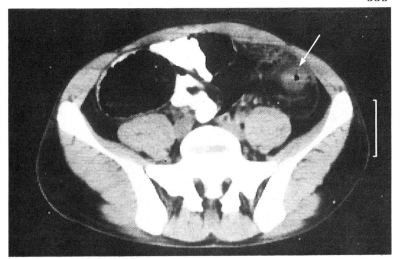

538

539

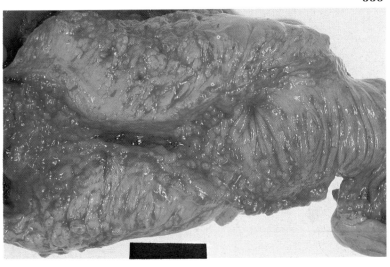

539 **Crohn's colitis.** The
colonic resection specimen
obtained from the same patient
as in **537** and **538**. The
descending colon is grossly
narrowed and there is fibrous
thickening of its wall. The
mucosa within and adjacent to
the stricture has a cobblestone
appearance. A small abscess
cavity (not shown) was also
identified within the wall of
this descending colon.

540

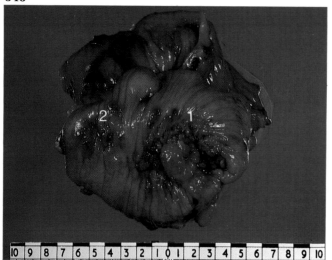

540 Crohn's disease. The ileo-caecal valve in this resection is distorted by hugely thickened folds of involved mucosa (1), leading to subacute obstruction at this site. In addition, a fistulous track (2) from the caecum 5 cm above the ileo-caecal valve (to its left in this picture) was found to be entering the terminal ileum.

541

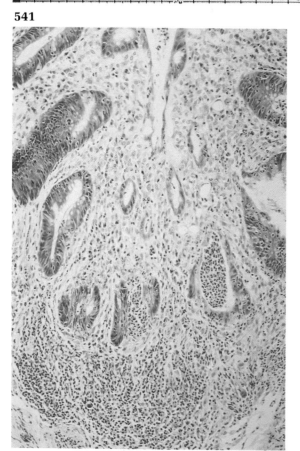

541 Crohn's colitis. The epithelium overlying a lymphoid aggregate shows acute inflammation with crypt abscesses and attenuation of the more superficial epithelium. This type of lesion, termed 'aphthoid ulcer', is said to be one of the earliest histological features of Crohn's disease.

542

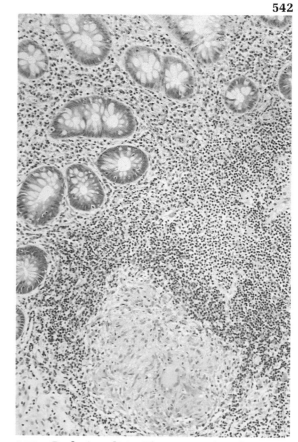

542 Crohn's colitis. The mucosal surface of this colonic biopsy is at the top of the field. In addition to chronic inflammation there is a granuloma at the bottom of the field; it includes a giant cell. This granuloma is better developed than is usual for Crohn's granulomas; neither foreign matter nor acid-fast bacilli were seen within it.

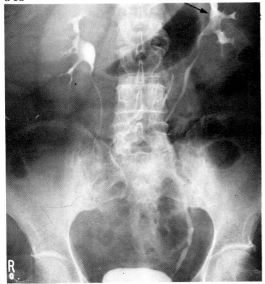

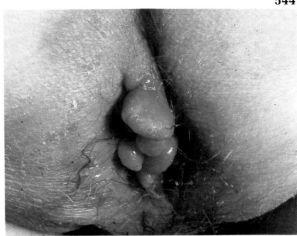

544   Perianal Crohn's disease. Abnormalities of the perianal region occur in about half of patients with Crohn's disease. The abnormalities range from simple asymptomatic skin tags to anal strictures, with perianal abscesses and fistula formation. In this example there are fleshy blue and pink skin tags with surrounding inflammation. An anal stricture was also present, precluding sigmoidoscopy.

543   Crohn's disease. An intravenous urogram was performed in this patient with Crohn's disease and renal colic. A calculus is seen within the left renal pelvis (arrow). Uric acid stones are a complication of Crohn's disease, especially in patients with an ileostomy, who tend to pass concentrated urine with a low pH. Furthermore, increased colonic oxalate absorption occurs in patients with steatorrhoea. Other renal complications of Crohn's disease include extrinsic ureteric compression from an inflammatory mass, rare renal amyloid and entero-vesical fistulae. This patient also has radiological evidence of sacro-ileitis.

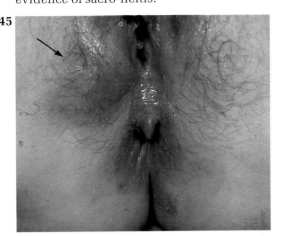

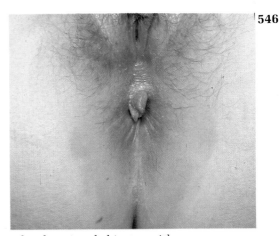

545 and 546   Perianal Crohn's disease. There is an inflamed red perianal skin tag with surrounding inflammation (**545**). Perineal sepsis has developed from a fistulous track from the anus into the perineum (arrow). The patient was treated with oral metronidazole for 4 weeks, leading to complete resolution of the inflammation, although the skin tags persist (**546**). Perianal Crohn's disease should be managed as conservatively as possible, and should not be treated if the patient is asymptomatic. Perianal inflammation and fistulae may be managed with metronidazole, whereas perianal abscesses may require incision and drainage under general anaesthesia.

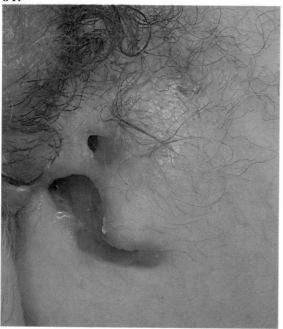

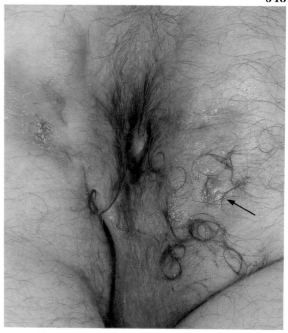

547   Perianal Crohn's disease. Deep cavitating perianal ulcers such as these may cause pain and may be complicated by perianal abscess formation or fistulae, or both. The penetrating abscesses may track forwards and involve the perineum. Severe perianal and perineal disease in association with active colonic Crohn's disease necessitated colectomy and ileostomy for this patient.

548   Perianal Crohn's disease. This patient had required multiple incisions and drainages of perianal abscesses. At the time of this photograph an abscess to the right of the anus had been discharging blood and pus intermittently.

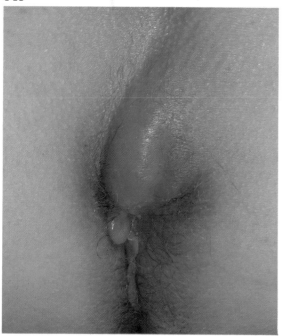

549   Perianal Crohn's disease. An acutely painful and tender perianal abscess has developed in this patient with otherwise quiescent Crohn's disease. Incision and drainage of the abscess was followed by complete recovery.

CHAPTER 13

Stomas

550 Ileostomy. A stoma is the surgical fixation of the opened bowel onto the anterior abdominal wall. The most common indication for a permanent ileostomy is in patients with ulcerative colitis or Crohn's disease undergoing pan-proctocolectomy. The ileostomy is covered with an appliance to collect the faecal effluent. Patients with ileostomy following pan-proctocolectomy have an almost normal life expectancy but run an increased risk of salt and water depletion, and of complications to the peristomal skin or the stoma itself. The figure shows a healthy ileostomy with surrounding pyoderma gangrenosum in a patient with a history of pan-proctocolectomy for Crohn's disease.

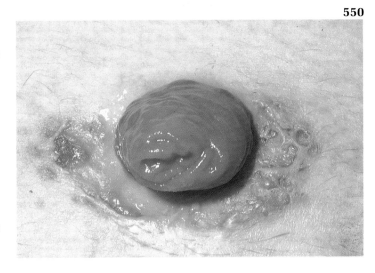

551 Colostomy. The most common indication for performing a colostomy is carcinoma of the rectum. Permanent colostomy is necessary in patients undergoing abdomino-perineal resection for low rectal tumours. A temporary colostomy may be fashioned electively in order to cover a distal anastomosis that may heal more safely in a defunctioned state. A temporary colostomy is routinely performed in the Hartmann's procedure, in which emergency resection of disease in the sigmoid colon is performed. Formation of stomas should be avoided where possible in the elderly and those with disabilities such as blindness or severe arthritis.

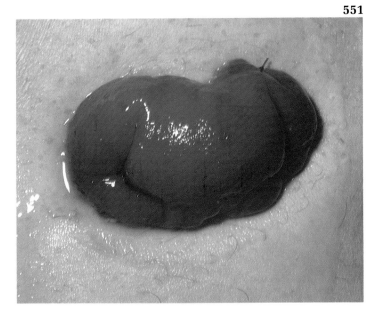

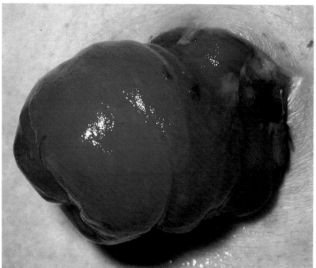

552 Prolapsed ileostomy. The stoma may prolapse and retract depending on posture, leading to leakage of stomal contents, particularly when the opening onto the abdominal wall is too large. Stomal reconstruction may become necessary.

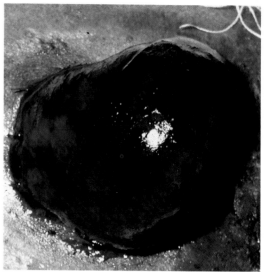

553 Colostomy ischaemia. End stomas may become ischaemic if the inferior mesenteric artery is ligated or if torsion or retraction of the ileo-colic artery develops. Venous congestion and darkening of the mucosa are present in this colostomy. Ileostomy ischaemia may develop from alternating prolapse and retraction causing damage to the small ileal mesenteric blood vessels.

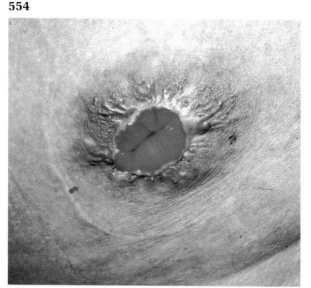

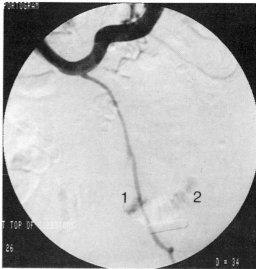

554 Peristomal varices. Patients with portal hypertension undergoing ileostomy or colostomy may develop portosystemic anastomoses via the veins of the anterior abdominal wall, leading to radiating venous collaterals around the stoma, as in this example.

555 Peristomal varices. A digital subtraction splenic venogram in a patient with bleeding via an ileostomy. There is a

collateral vessel between the splenic vein and the anterior abdominal wall around the site of the ileostomy. A bleeding point has been demonstrated (1) and contrast is pooling retrogradely into the bowel from the stoma (2). Bleeding from peristomal varices is a particular problem in patients with primary sclerosing cholangitis and ulcerative colitis after pan-proctocolectomy and the formation of a permanent ileostomy.

CHAPTER 14

Perianal Disorders

556   Haemorrhoids. These are varices of the superior haemorrhoidal vein that drain into the inferior mesenteric vein. Most haemorrhoids occur in otherwise healthy people, but may be precipitated or aggravated by pregnancy, pelvic tumours and recurrent straining in patients with chronic constipation. Rectal bleeding is the usual presenting symptom. In this unusual view the flexible sigmoidoscope has been inverted within the rectum to show the anorectal junction and haemorrhoids within the anal canal. Patients presenting with rectal bleeding who are found to have haemorrhoids should undergo rigid or flexible sigmoidoscopy to exclude a lesion higher up in the colon or rectum. The haemorrhoids should not be assumed to be the cause of the bleeding unless a higher lesion has been excluded. Asymptomatic haemorrhoids, although presenting with minor haemorrhage, may not require specific treatment. Injection sclerotherapy via a proctoscope is the conventional method of treatment for small symptomatic haemorrhoids.

556

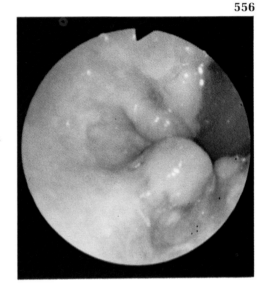

557   Prolapsed haemorrhoids. Moderate or large haemorrhoids commonly prolapse on defecation and reduce spontaneously or may be replaced digitally by the patient. Large haemorrhoids may remain persistently prolapsed outside the anal canal. The figure is a severe example of prolapsed haemorrhoids, with superficial ulceration and mucosal congestion. Recurrent or permanent prolapse may be an indication for haemorrhoidectomy.

557

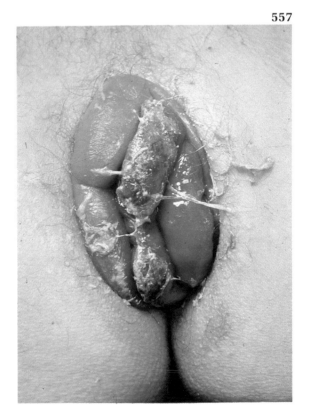

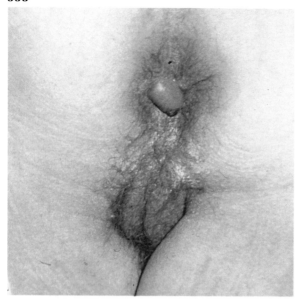

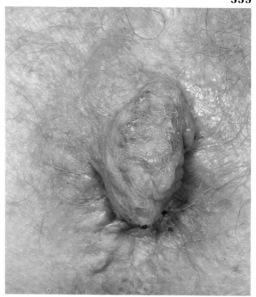

558 Thrombosed haemorrhoids. This phenomenon may occur when prolapsed haemorrhoids are trapped by the anal sphincter, leading to venous occlusion and thrombosis. The prolapsed haemorrhoids are purple in colour and are very tender. Thrombosed haemorrhoids may fibrose completely with spontaneous cure. Some patients with thrombosed haemorrhoids require hospital admission for bed rest, pain relief and local compresses. The timing of operative intervention in these patients is controversial.

559 Haemorrhoidal varices. The superior haemorrhoidal vessels are one of the sites of anastomosis between the portal and systemic venous systems. Patients with portal hypertension are at risk for developing large haemorrhoidal varices, as in this example. Recurrent and extensive haemorrhages may occur, necessitating a porta-systemic shunt. Injection sclerotherapy should not normally be attempted.

560

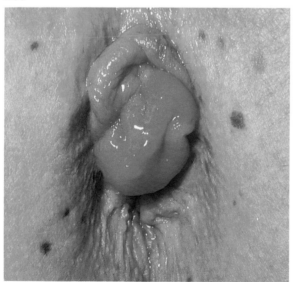

560 Rectal prolapse. Rectal prolapse may be complete or incomplete. In this example part of the rectal mucosa has prolapsed a few inches from the anal verge. Partial mucosal prolapse is often associated with haemorrhoids. Treatment of partial prolapse in adults may include a submucosal sclerosant injection, or haemorrhoidectomy with excision of the redundant mucosa. Constipation may require therapy with laxatives or bulking agents.

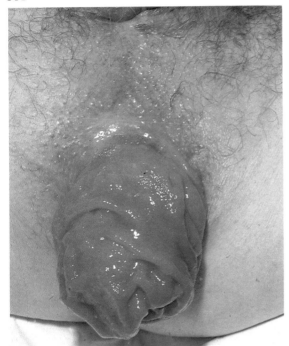

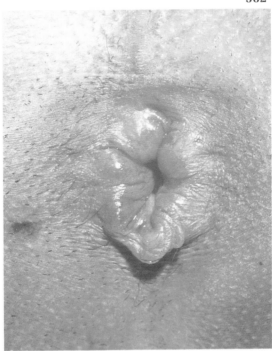

561 Rectal prolapse. Complete prolapse of all layers of the rectal wall usually occurs in elderly females. Prolapse may be recurrent or permanent. There may be associated incontinence of faeces due to the stretching of the anal sphincter and mucus discharge from the prolapsed bowel. A variety of operative methods are available for treating complete rectal prolapse. The rectum may require fixation within the pelvic cavity by means of an abdominal operation.

562 Anal fissure. Single or multiple tears of the anal skin usually result from the passage of a large constipated stool. Acute anal pain and superficial bleeding may result. Spasm of the anal sphincter may lead to a vicious circle of worsening constipation and failure of the fissure to heal. Local anaesthetic creams are normally prescribed, but intractable cases may require operative stretching of the anal sphincter under general anaesthetic.

563 Fistula-in-ano. This term is given to fistulae or sinuses lying between the perianal skin and the anorectal mucosa. Fistula and sinus formation may result from subcutaneous or submucosal abscesses from infected anal glands. Fistulae-in-ano are usually idiopathic, but they may complicate perianal Crohn's disease or tuberculosis. Occasionally they are a presenting feature of rectal carcinoma. The fistula usually presents with pain, or recurrent discharge of pus or sero-sanguinous material. Operative exploration and laying open of the fistula may be necessary. Patients with Crohn's disease and fistula-in-ano should be managed conservatively with metronidazole and operative drainage of any perianal abscess.

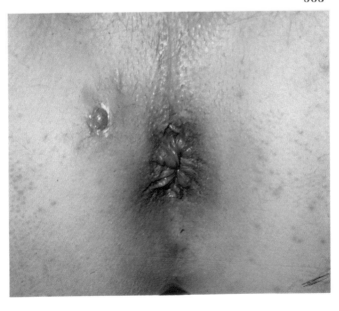

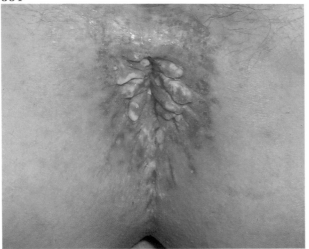

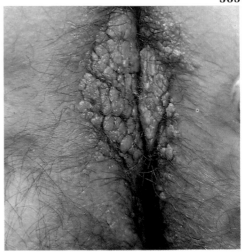

564   Pruritus ani. The figure shows extensive lichenification of the perianal skin, due to recurrent pruritus ani. There are a number of possible causes of pruritus ani, including poor local hygiene, leakage of mucus from haemorrhoids, proctitis, rectal neoplasms or threadworm infestation. Fungal infections may supervene. Any underlying cause should be treated. The pruritus itself may respond to local corticosteroid creams and attention to local hygiene.

565   Perianal condylomata. These warts, also known as condylomata acuminata, are common in homosexual men. They are pedunculated growths that occur in the perianal region and within the anal canal. The human papilloma virus has been implicated in this disease. Approaches to treatment include topical podophyllin, electrocautery, cryotherapy or scissor excision. Repeated treatment is often necessary. Excision biopsy may be necessary to exclude squamous carcinoma.

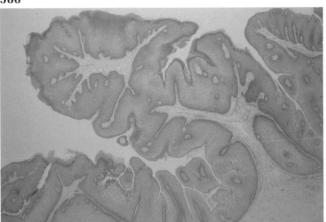

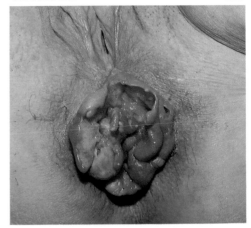

566   Perianal warts. The epithelium of this anus reflects the morphological features of a wart virus infection. Epithelial thickening (acanthosis) and papillomatosis are seen over a wide area.

567   Anal carcinoma. Anal carcinoma may present with pruritus ani, perianal warts or fissures. Radical excision of the anus, rectum and perianal skin, together with block dissection of the inguinal lymph nodes and the formation of a permanent colostomy, is the operation of choice. Radiotherapy is indicated for small carcinomas with low-grade malignancy on histological examination, and in treating recurrent disease.

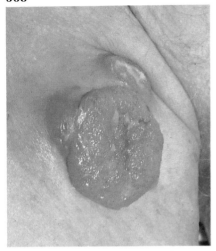

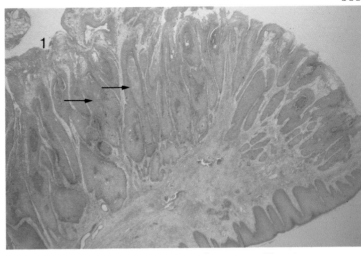

568 Anal carcinoma. Anal carcinoma differs from carcinoma of the rectum in its lymphatic drainage. Secondary inguinal lymph node deposits may be the presenting feature in a small number of patients. In this example the lymph nodes have ulcerated through the skin and fungated.

569 Anal carcinoma. A section from an infiltrating, moderately differentiated squamous cell carcinoma of the anus. Non-neoplastic squamous epithelium is seen at the bottom right and carcinoma is seen above. There is ulceration of the surface of the tumour (1), and red-staining islands of keratin are present underneath (arrows).

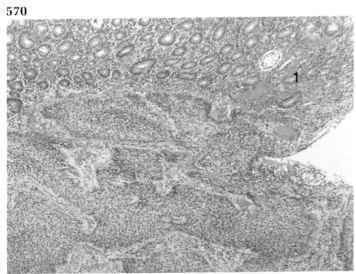

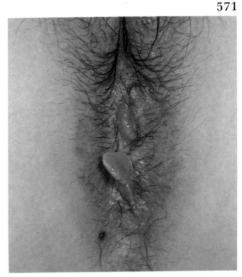

570 Anal carcinoma. A section from a basiloid carcinoma at the junction of rectum (1) and anus. In this type of tumour the cells are smaller and more basophilic than in squamous carcinoma. This tumour is considered to arise from anal transitional epithelium, or cloacal rests. This tumour is more aggressive than its cutaneous counterpart (basal cell carcinoma). It behaves at least as aggressively as squamous cell carcinoma; indeed, areas of squamous differentiation may be seen within it.

571 Perianal skin tags. This common abnormality may follow a perianal haematoma or thrombosis and strangulation of haemorrhoids. They may be complicated by the features of anal fissure and associated constipation. The presence of perianal skin tags should alert the attending physician to the possibility of Crohn's disease, as more than 50% of patients with Crohn's disease of the colon have some form of perianal lesion. Small violaceous perianal skin tags are seen in this young woman with Crohn's colitis.

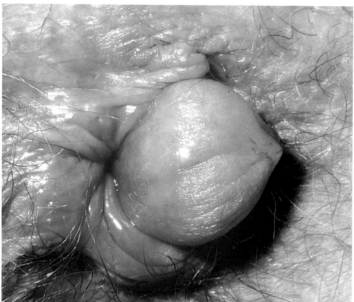 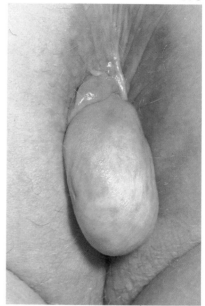

572 and **573** **Fibro-epithelial polyps.** Recurrent prolapsing haemorrhoids may scar and become fibrosed. This fibrotic nodule may prolapse with continued straining, so that it eventually passes outside the anal canal, requiring manual replacement after defecation. It may remain permanently prolapsed, as is the case in **573**.

574

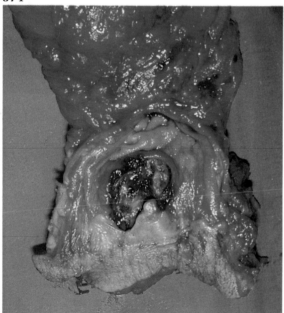

574 **Malignant melanoma.** A malignant melanoma at the anal margin is relatively rare, and it carries a poor prognosis despite radical resection. Secondary deposits may be found in bowel (**344**).

CHAPTER 15

Gastrointestinal Infections

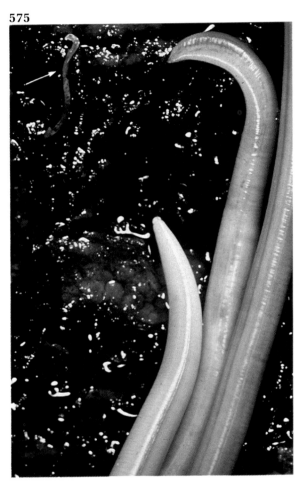

575

575 Worm infections. The nematode *Ascaris lumbricoides* (roundworm) and the much smaller hookworm (*Ankylostoma duodenale*, arrow) are seen lying within the intestine at post-mortem. Hookworm infection is common in the Third World countries, but only heavy infections are clinically important. Hookworm infection can lead to anaemia and hypoalbuminaemia. The larvae enter the body through intact skin and traverse the lungs, and the adults emerge in the proximal jejunum. The diagnosis is made by finding ova in the faeces or adult worms in the duodenal or jejunal fluid.

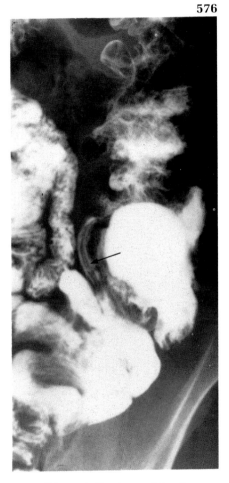

576

576 Worm infections. A barium meal and follow-through examination has identified a roundworm in the terminal ileum (arrow). Roundworm infections are often asymptomatic, but occasionally large numbers of adult worms may form a bolus and cause intestinal obstruction. The diagnosis is normally made by finding ova in the faeces, although occasionally adult worms are passed per rectum. Treatment with albendozole, mebendazole or one of the piperazine compounds eliminates the infection.

201

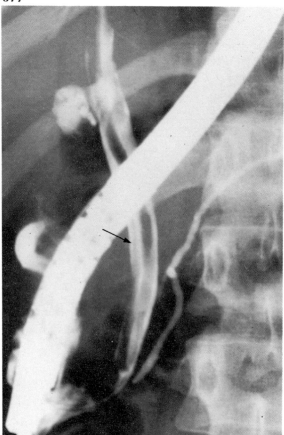

577 Worm infections. A roundworm is outlined
with contrast in the common bile duct at
endoscopic retrograde cholangiography (arrow).
Roundworms occasionally cause common bile
duct or pancreatic duct obstruction.

578

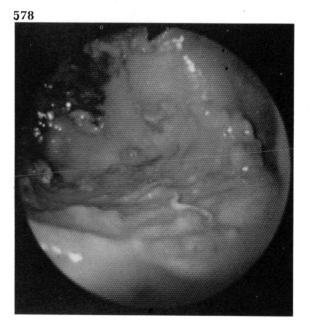

578 Threadworm infestation. A threadworm
(*Enterobius vermicularis*) is seen in the rectum
during colonoscopy. Threadworms may cause
severe pruritus ani. Their ova may be detected by
microscopic examination of a piece of adhesive
tape placed on the perianal skin.

579 Threadworm infestation. A transverse section of a threadworm is seen in the upper part of the field near to normal appendiceal mucosa. The presence of these worms is a coincidence, and not associated with disease of the appendix.

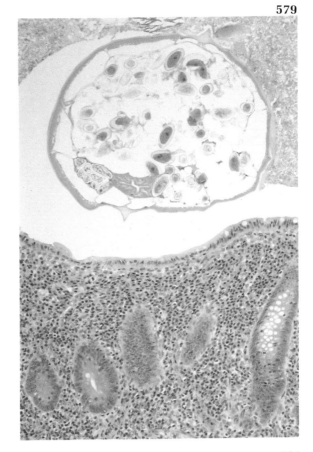

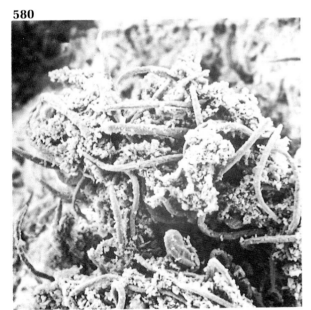

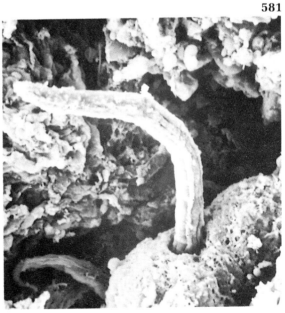

580 and **581 Strongyloidiasis.** *Strongyloides stercoralis* infections are seen most commonly in South-East Asia and West Africa. The usual symptoms are those of malabsorption and mild abdominal distension. Patients with strongyloidiasis may remain asymptomatic for many years. The most serious consequence of strongyloidiasis is the hyperinfection syndrome that occurs in immunosuppressed patients (including those recently commenced on corticosteroids). **580** is a scanning electron micrograph of a mass of these worms covering the intestinal epithelial surface. One of them can be seen entering the intestinal crypt in a higher-magnification view in **581**.

582

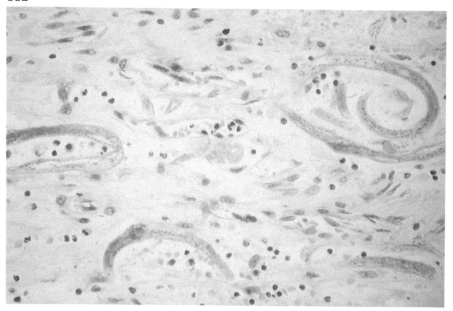

582 Strongyloidiasis. This section shows several worms in the submucosa of the small intestine of a patient with overwhelming *Strongyloides* hyperinfection following immunosuppression for renal transplantation.

583

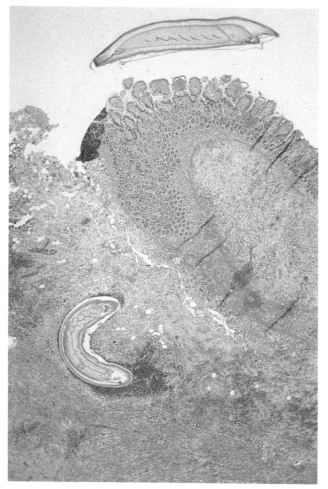

583 Ileal anisakiasis. Anisakiasis is an infection caused by the larvae of nematodes belonging to the family Anisakidae. The majority of patients with this infection present with epigastric pain, nausea or vomiting 12–24 h after eating infected fish. There may be haematemesis during the acute stage of the disease. In this section one larva is lying within the ileal lumen and another has penetrated the ileal wall, causing inflammation and ulceration. The incidence of this infection is highest in Japan, followed by The Netherlands, Scandinavia and South America.

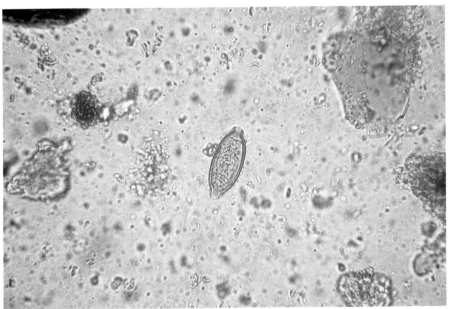

584 Trichuriasis. Infection with this nematode worm can lead to colitis. The diagnosis is made by finding the characteristic barrel-shaped eggs in the faeces. A *Trichuris Trichiura* egg is seen in the centre of the photograph of a formol–ether stool concentrate.

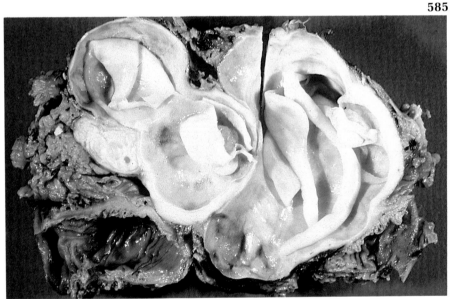

585 Hydatid disease. This cestode infection occurs in many different parts of the world, including Europe, North America, the USSR, Japan, and northern and eastern Africa. The liver and lungs are the most common organs affected by this parasite. It may be contracted by handling dogs or sheep with contaminated hair, or by consuming contaminated vegetables or water. Hydatid cysts may occur in the mesentery, as in this photograph. Patients may present with a palpable mass or pain due to pressure from enlarging cysts in the liver. Rupture of a hydatid cyst into the peritoneal cavity may cause peritonitis or occasionally an acute anaphylactic reaction. Treatment consists of careful surgical excision of the cyst, taking care not to rupture the cyst fluid into the peritoneal cavity, as scolices within the fluid usually implant elsewhere, leading to recurrent disease.

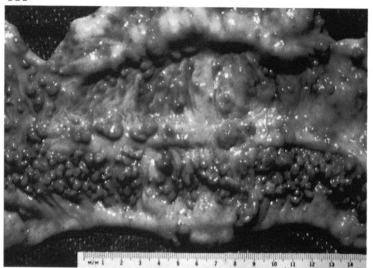

586 Schistosomiasis. The usual member of this family of trematodes to affect the gastrointestinal tract is *Schistosoma mansoni*. The cercariae are normally liberated by snails into fresh water, penetrate intact skin, and migrate via the bloodstream to the lungs and liver. Adult worms reside in the inferior mesenteric vein, where they produce large numbers of ova that are retained within the wall of the colon. The ova then migrate through into the bowel wall and lead to a colitis. This is a gross example of *S. mansoni* colitis with polyp formation. Histological examination of these polyps will demonstrate the ova. Praziquantel is the treatment of choice.

587

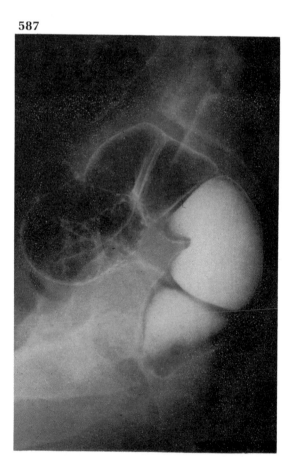

588

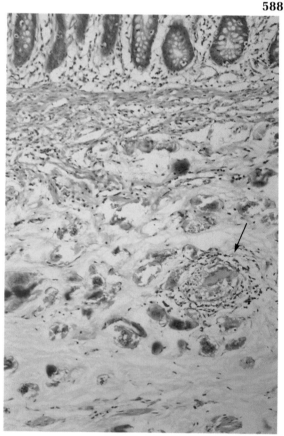

587 Schistosomiasis. A lateral view of the rectum and recto-sigmoid colon in a patient with *S. mansoni* colitis. Granularity and superficial ulceration of the mucosa of the sigmoid colon are shown. The rectum itself is usually spared.

588 Schistosomiasis. Section of mucosa and submucosa from a Malawian patient with schistosomiasis. Many calcified and degenerate ova are seen in the lower part of the photograph. One of the ova has stimulated a granulomatous reaction (arrow).

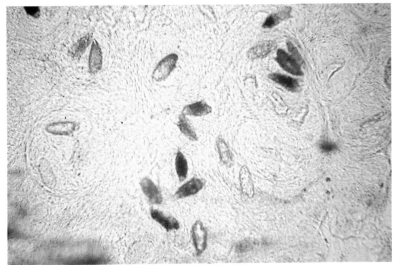

589 Schistosomiasis. A useful method for making a rapid diagnosis of *S. mansoni* is to press snips of rectal mucosa between glass slides and examine them immediately under a microscope. The ova of *S. mansoni* are seen in this unstained smear.

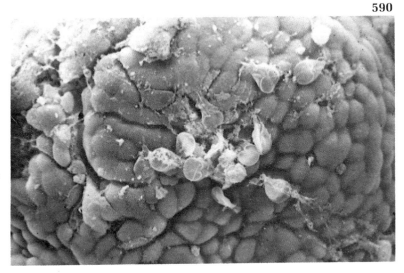

590 Giardiasis. This protozoan parasite can infest the small intestine and lead to a variety of clinical presentations, including acute (travellers') diarrhoea or chronic malabsorption. The parasite *Giardia lamblia* exists worldwide, and infections usually arise from contaminated water. Several epidemics have occurred in Europe and the USA. This scanning electron micrograph shows trophozoites of *G. lamblia* residing on the tip of a jejunal villus.

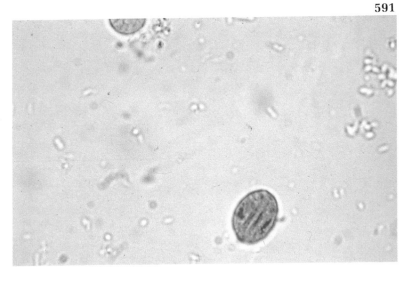

591 Giardiasis. *Giardia* cysts are seen on iodine staining of a wet preparation of fresh faeces. This is the usual method of diagnosis, but jejunal aspiration and biopsy may be necessary as multiple stool examinations may fail to yield the organism.

592

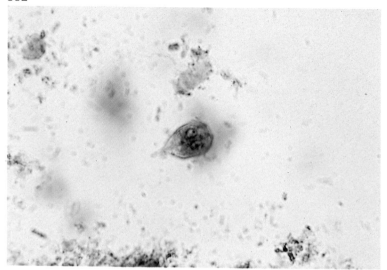

592 Giardiasis. A trophozoite of *Giardia lamblia* has been identified by iron haematoxylin staining of a wet preparation of faeces. Giardiasis is eliminated by treatment with metronidazole or tinidazole.

593

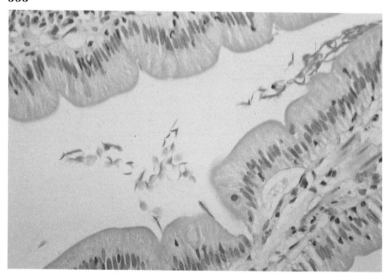

593 Giardiasis. A duodenal biopsy showing numerous *Giardia lamblia* trophozoites. These are seen as purplish flakes partly adherent to the villous epithelium.

594

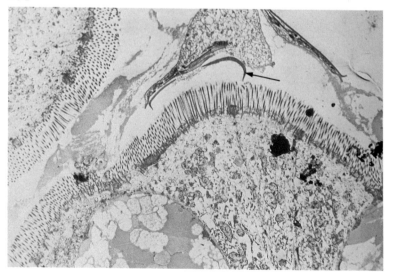

594 Giardiasis. Transmission electron micrograph of the same case as **593**. A trophozoite (arrow) adheres to the microvillous enterocyte border.

595 and **596** **Cryptosporidiosis.**
This coccidian parasite is now
recognised as a common cause of
self-limiting acute diarrhoea,
particularly in children.
Immunocompromised patients,
particularly those with the
acquired immune deficiency
syndrome (AIDS), are at risk of
fatal infection with this parasite,
leading to a profuse secretory
diarrhoea, with profound
malabsorption and weight loss.
The diagnosis is made by
demonstration of the parasite in
intestinal biopsies or in the
stools. The auramine method
(**595**) or a modified Ziehl–
Neelsen technique (**596**) may be
used for parasite identification.
Drug treatment of this infection
has proved generally
unsuccessful.

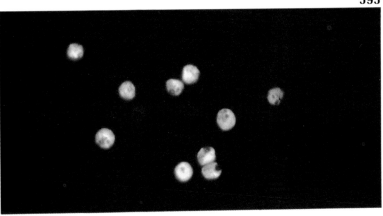

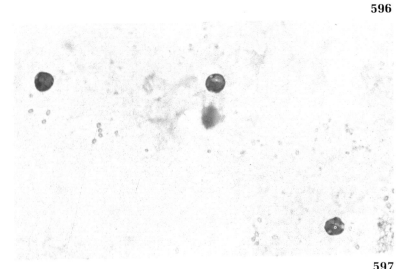

596

597

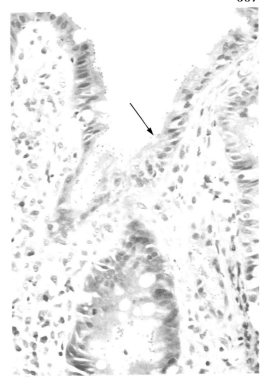

597 **Cryptosporidiosis.** A rectal biopsy from a patient
with acquired immune deficiency syndrome.
Numerous darkly staining particles are seen on the
luminal border of the glandular and more superficial
epithelium (arrow). These are cryptosporidia. The
lamina propria shows a little chronic inflammation.

598

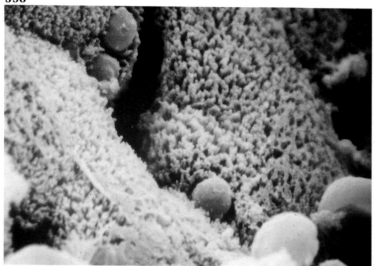

598 Cryptosporidiosis.
Scanning electron microscopy shows spherical cryptosporidia lying on and partly within the surface of the intestinal epithelium.

599

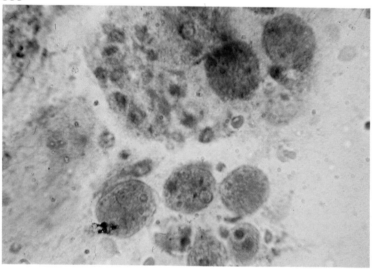

599 Amoebiasis. Colonic infection with *Entamoeba histolytica* is an important cause of colitis, especially in tropical regions where sanitation is poor. Sporadic cases may occur in the West. Amoebic colitis must be differentiated from ulcerative colitis or Crohn's disease. The diagnosis is made by finding the characteristic motile amoebae with their ingested red cells during microscopy of a fresh stool specimen (as here) after iron haematoxylin staining. The condition is treated with metronidazole or tinidazole.

600

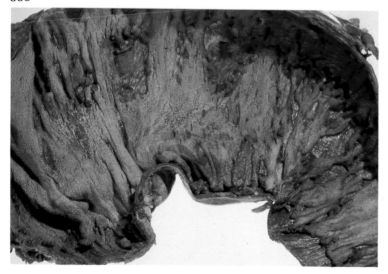

600 Amoebic colitis. A postmortem photograph of the colonic mucosal surface in a patient with amoebic colitis. Several 'punched out' ulcers with haemorrhagic edges can be seen.

601 Amoebic colitis. At least four pale-staining amoebae (arrow) are embedded within slough adjacent to ulcerated and inflamed large bowel epithelium on the right.

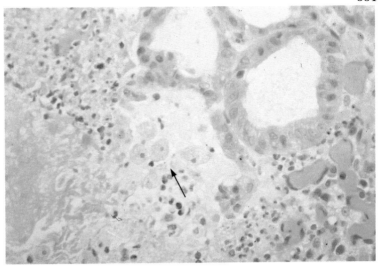

602 Amoebic liver abscess (arrow) may occur in the absence of overt colonic infection, or may present many years after an episode of colitis. Pleuritic-type chest pain or right upper quadrant pain and tenderness are the usual presenting features. Occasionally the abscess may enlarge and rupture through the diaphragm into the right pleural cavity or lung. Amoebic abscesses are a cause of fever of unknown origin. This computerised tomographic scan has demonstrated a single amoebic abscess in the right lobe of the liver.

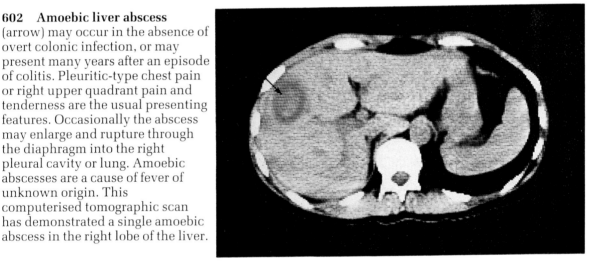

603 Amoebiasis. Amoebic liver abscesses normally respond to oral metronidazole therapy. Diloxanide furoate should also be given to eradicate chronic intestinal infections in patients with liver abscesses. Sometimes large abscesses may warrant percutaneous aspiration, which yields the characteristic reddish-brown pus that may contain amoebae. The appearance of this pus has been likened to anchovy sauce.

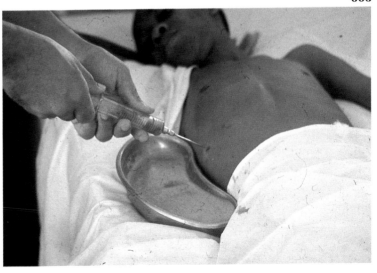

604

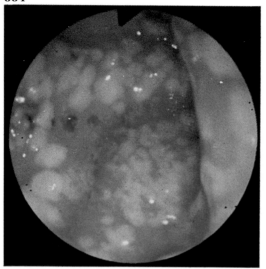

604 Pseudomembranous colitis. This form of colitis is characterised by confluent colonic inflammation with pseudomembrane formation. This colonoscopic view illustrates the greenish pseudomembrane overlying the inflamed mucosal surface. It is now known that *Clostridium difficile* and its heat-labile toxin are the cause of this colitis. The disease is usually preceded by broad-spectrum antibiotic therapy. The diagnosis is made using commercially available techniques for the identification of the toxin in the faeces, or by culture of the organisms. The standard treatment of pseudomembranous colitis is oral vancomycin, although metronidazole is cheaper and may be equally effective.

605

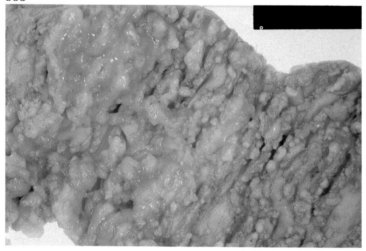

605 Pseudomembranous colitis. A post-mortem view of part of the colon from a patient with pseudomembranous colitis. Irregular ulceration is seen leaving islands of surviving epithelium and a covering of mucopus (centre field and upper left). The green colour in this picture is an accurate reflection of the mucosal appearance of pseudomembranous colitis in life.

606

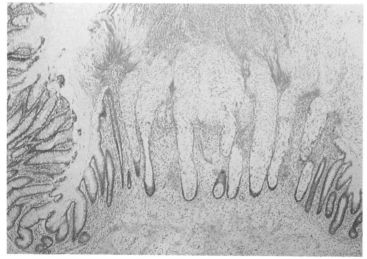

606 Pseudomembranous colitis. The characteristic histological feature is the 'summit' lesion—the surface spray of fibrin and pus from the superficial lamina propria. Several of these summit lesions have coalesced in this field to produce composite destruction of epithelium that can lead to complete ulceration. In this field the fibrin appears as red plumes in the upper centre: the subjacent mucosa and submucosa are oedematous and inflamed. Another feature of this condition is the relative normality of the epithelium seen to either side of the diseased area.

607 Typhoid fever. This infection is endemic in most tropical countries, and it is caused by Gram-negative bacilli of the *Salmonella* genus. Occasional epidemics occur in the West. Symptoms develop approximately 2 weeks after the ingestion of infected food. Fever, general malaise and bradycardia are seen in the first week, and a macular rash may develop over the trunk, as in this patient. Blood cultures are useful in making an early diagnosis. Treatment with chloramphenicol or cotrimoxazole is essential to prevent life-threatening intestinal haemorrhage or severe toxaemia.

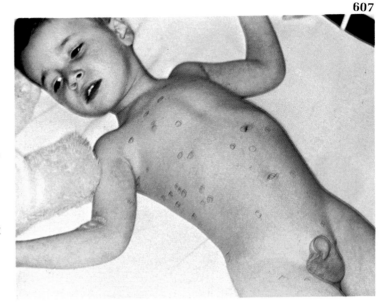

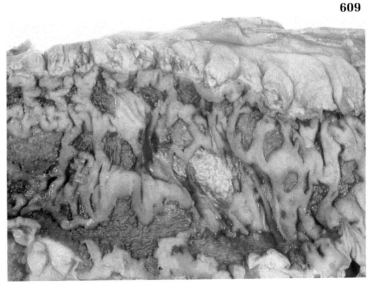

608 Typhoid fever. A fixed specimen of ileum, illustrating the enlarged Peyer's patches of lymphoid tissue that characterise this disorder. Ileal perforation or haemorrhage may occur in the third week of the illness.

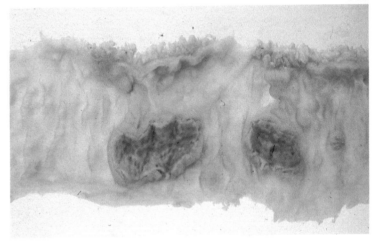

609 *Salmonella* enterocolitis. This is the mucosal surface of a colectomy specimen from a patient with fulminating colitis. Deep ulcers had penetrated through the submucosa into muscle.

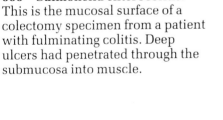

610

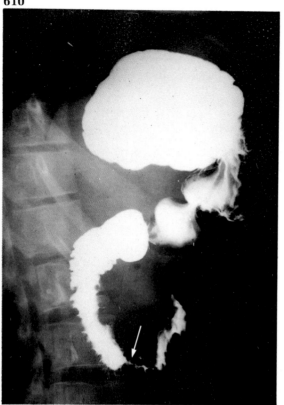

610 Intestinal tuberculosis. This disease is common in Third World countries, particularly India and South-East Asia. Occasional cases are seen in Europe and North America. The infection is usually secondary to pulmonary tuberculosis, being caused by the ingestion of *Mycobacterium tuberculosis* from the sputum into the stomach and intestine. Infection with *M. bovis* may be seen in those who have consumed unpasteurised milk. Any part of the gastrointestinal tract may be involved, but the small intestine usually bears the brunt of the infection. This barium meal examination has shown stricturing and ulceration of the third and fourth parts of the duodenum (arrow). Intestinal tuberculosis is often difficult to diagnose, and laparoscopy or laparotomy may be necessary to obtain tissue for histological examination. Endoscopic biopsy may yield the typical caseating granulomata with acid-fast bacilli on Ziehl–Neelsen staining.

611

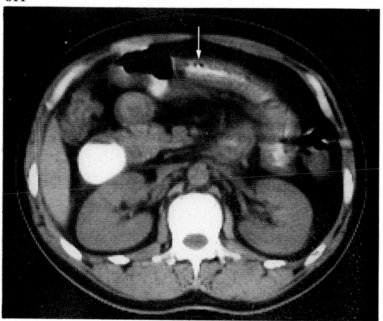

611 Intestinal tuberculosis. Computerised tomography in intestinal tuberculosis may show thickened loops of small intestine, peritoneal seedlings or mesenteric lymphadenopathy. This computerised tomographic scan has shown thickening of a loop of small intestine that contains orally administered contrast (arrow).

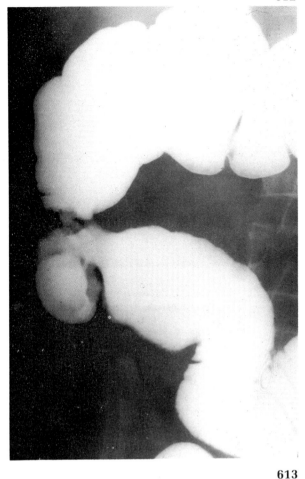

612   Intestinal tuberculosis. This barium study has demonstrated stricturing and ulceration of the terminal ileum and caecum due to tuberculosis. Intestinal tuberculosis must be differentiated from lymphoma, Crohn's disease or ischaemia. Complications of tuberculosis of the gut include intestinal haemorrhage or obstruction, and tuberculous peritonitis with ascites. Once the diagnosis has been established, antituberculous therapy must be given for at least 9 months.

613   Intestinal tuberculosis. The ileocaecal junction of a patient with intestinal tuberculosis. The pale mass in the upper right of the field is a caseous lymph node, and the ileum is ulcerated just below this (arrow).

614

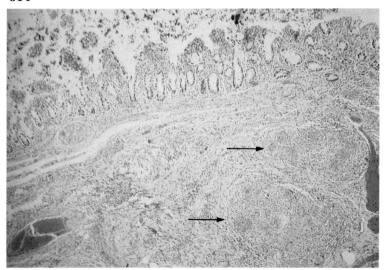

614 Intestinal tuberculosis. A histological section of the ileal ulcer seen in **613**. The epithelium shows chronic inflammation and erosion. Submucosal granulomas are seen on the right (arrows).

615

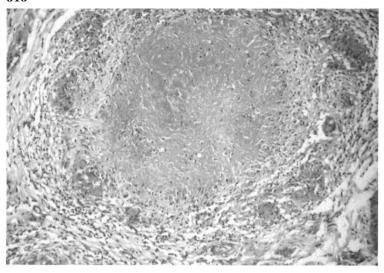

615 and **616   Intestinal tuberculosis.** A submucosal granuloma showing central caseous necrosis with occasional giant cells is seen in **615**. The adjacent submucosa is infiltrated by chronic inflammatory cells. Ziehl–Neelsen staining (**616**) shows the characteristic histological morphology of *Mycobacterium tuberculosis*. High magnification using an oil immersion lens has demonstrated a red-staining tubercle bacillus.

616

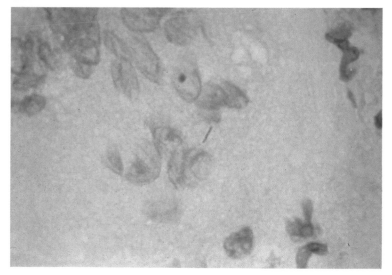

617

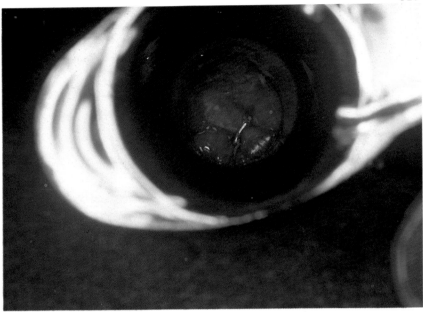

617 Gonorrhoea. A proctoscopic view of the rectal mucosa in a patient with gonorrhoea. Rectal infection with *Neisseria gonorrhoeae* may be asymptomatic or may lead to perianal discharge, bleeding or pruritus ani. The rectal mucosa is inflamed and oedematous, with confluent areas of muco-pus. Proctoscopic abnormalities are usually confined to the lower 10cm of rectal mucosa. To make the diagnosis, a swab is passed through the proctoscope and the mucus is examined microscopically or cultured on selective media. Gonorrhoeal infection of the rectum usually results from receptive anal intercourse and is most commonly seen in male homosexuals.

618

618 Syphilis. A photograph of the anus with the perianal chancres of primary syphilis resulting from receptive anal intercourse. This infection is due to the spirochaetal bacterium *Treponema pallidum*. Unlike primary chancres of the external genitalia, perianal lesions are often painful and friable. Symptoms of proctitis may follow syphilis of the rectum. The diagnosis of primary syphilis is made by dark-ground microscopy of exudate obtained from the base of one of these chancres. If the spirochaete is not identified by this method, serological tests for syphilis such as the *T. pallidum* haemagglutination test may be employed.

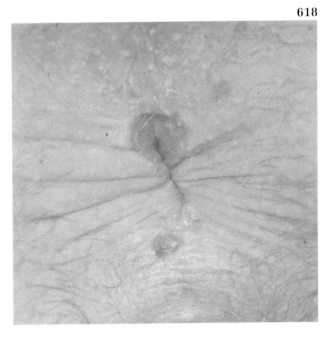

619

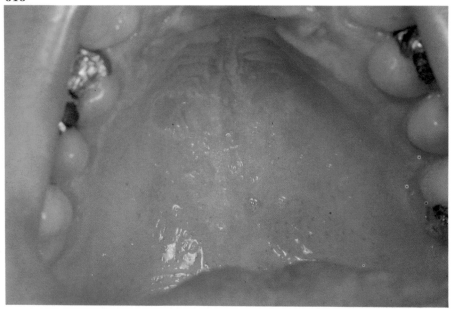

620

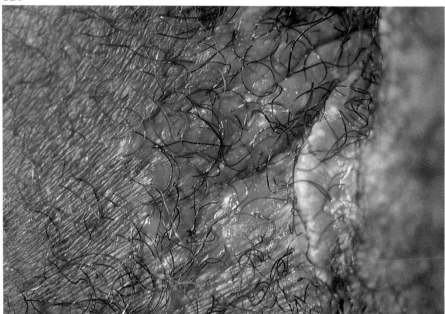

619 and **620** **Syphilis.** Secondary syphilis occurs about 6 weeks after an untreated primary infection, and is manifested by a macular rash, painless greyish-white erosions of the oral mucosa (**619**) and occasionally condylomata lata (warty infiltration of the perianal skin shown in **620**). Both of these lesions are highly infectious.

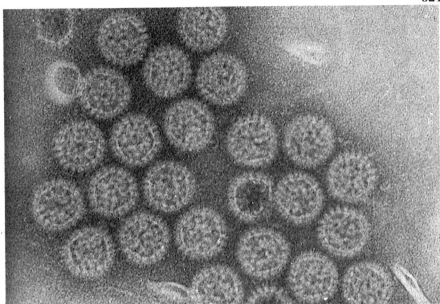

621 Viral gastroenteritis. This electron micrograph of a stool sample illustrates the rotavirus. This virus is responsible for approximately 80% of infant admissions to hospital with gastroenteritis. The virus has a diameter of 65–70 nm.

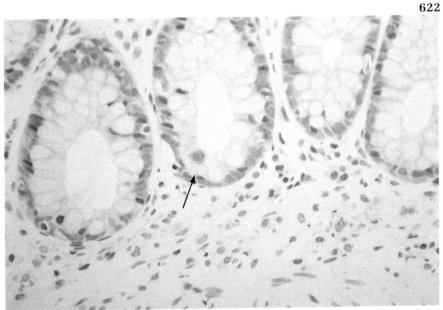

622 Acquired immune deficiency syndrome (AIDS). This increasingly common disease is caused by the human immunodeficiency virus (HIV). Transmission occurs sexually or from administration of infected blood or blood products. This virus replicates in helper T-lymphocytes, leading to profound depression of the cell-mediated immune response. The presence of certain opportunistic infections or Kaposi's sarcoma in a patient with serological evidence of HIV infection confirms that the full AIDS syndrome has developed. This rectal biopsy was obtained from a patient with AIDS. One epithelial cell of the crypt (arrow) contains a large nucleus and a prominent eosinophilic nucleolus, indicating cytomegalovirus infection of the rectum.

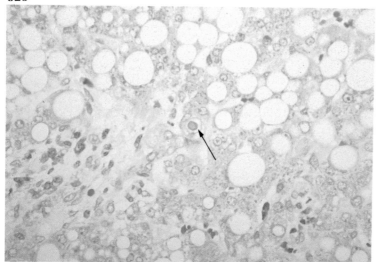

623 Acquired immune deficiency syndrome. This liver biopsy section has been stained by the Giemsa method. There is fatty change, and a hepatocyte shows a large nucleus with a prominent nucleolus indicative of cytomegalovirus infection (arrow).

624

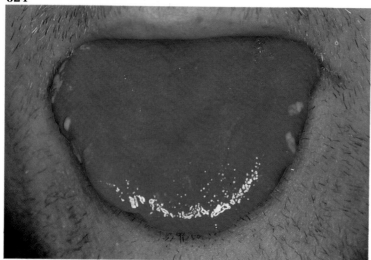

624 Acquired immune deficiency syndrome. There are white plaques of candida on the tongue of this male homosexual with AIDS. Oral candidiasis is common in patients with HIV infection (see **47**) but does not in itself mean that the patient has AIDS. Oesophageal candidiasis is often present in patients with oral candidiasis (see **48** to **50**). An HIV antibody-positive patient with oesophageal candidiasis is deemed to have the full AIDS syndrome.

625

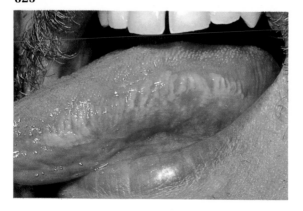

625 Acquired immune deficiency syndrome. These greyish-white lesions on the lateral borders of the tongue are termed hairy leucoplakia. Histological examination reveals keratin projections resembling hairs. This is probably due to a virus infection.

626 and **627** **Kaposi's sarcoma.** These tumours arise from vascular endothelium. They rarely occur in patients under the age of 60 years in the absence of HIV infection. **626** shows a vascular tumour of the palate, and **627** illustrates a similar lesion of the rectal mucosa. Kaposi's sarcoma may occur virtually anywhere in the gastrointestinal tract. Its presence indicates that a patient with HIV infection has the fully developed AIDS syndrome.

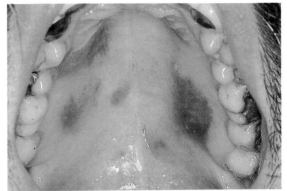

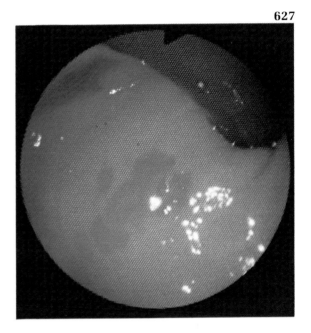
627

628 **Kaposi's sarcoma.** A photograph of a Kaposi's sarcoma on the lateral chest wall of a young male homosexual with AIDS. The plaque of bluish discolouration is 2 cm in diameter and there is surrounding infiltration. Kaposi's sarcomata may occur anywhere on the skin, but typically involve the trunk, arms or face. The tumours usually enlarge slowly, but may be rapidly progressive and may ulcerate. They are malignant, but rarely life-threatening, as AIDS patients with Kaposi's sarcoma usually die from opportunistic infections.

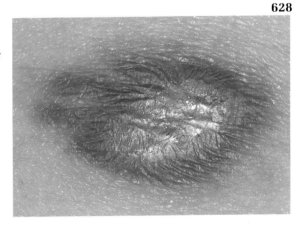
628

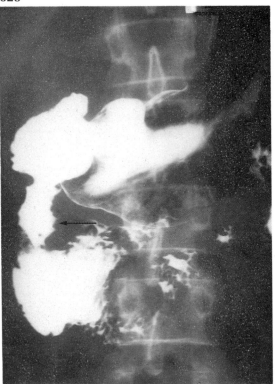

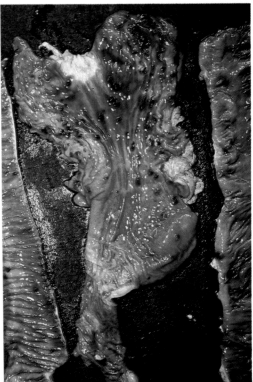

629   Kaposi's sarcoma. A barium meal in a patient with AIDS presenting with symptoms of high intestinal obstruction. The second part of the duodenum is narrowed due to a Kaposi's sarcoma (arrow). Other complications from gastrointestinal Kaposi's sarcomas include ulceration, haemorrhage and diarrhoea. Cryptosporidia may be a cause of diarrhoea and weight loss in patients with AIDS (see **595** to **598**).

630   Kaposi's sarcoma. A post-mortem has been performed on an African patient with AIDS. There are multiple vascular Kaposi's sarcomas of the stomach and colon. Post-mortem studies have shown that more than 70% of patients with Kaposi's sarcomas of the skin have tumours within the gastrointestinal tract.

631

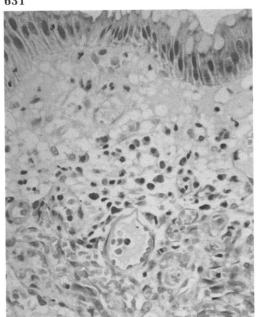

631   Acquired immune deficiency syndrome.
A gastric biopsy of a patient with AIDS. The superficial foveolar epithelium is seen at the top of the field. There is a tangled network of vascular spaces lined by neoplastic spindle-shaped cells, due to infiltration by Kaposi's sarcoma. This preparation is stained with phloxine-tartrazine.

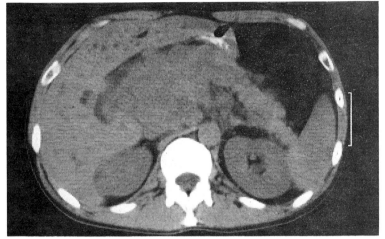

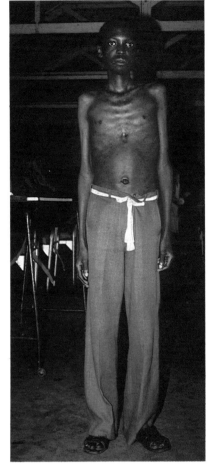

632 Acquired immune deficiency syndrome. A computerised tomographic scan of the upper abdomen of a patient with AIDS and a rapidly enlarging painful mass in the upper abdomen. The whole of the central portion of the abdomen is occupied by the mass of mesenteric lymph nodes infiltrated by a non-Hodgkin's lymphoma. These tumours are resistant to therapy and mean survival is less than 1 year.

633 Acquired immune deficiency syndrome. This is a Ugandan man with enteropathic AIDS ('slim' disease). African patients with enteropathic AIDS present with severe weight loss and diarrhoea, often due to cryptosporidiosis.

634 Acquired immune deficiency syndrome. Another infection that is common in patients with AIDS is that due to *Isospora belli*. Infection with this coccidian parasite may lead to abdominal pain, diarrhoea and weight loss. Diagnosis is made by examination of formol-ether concentrates of stool. A freshly passed oocyst is seen in the centre of the field.

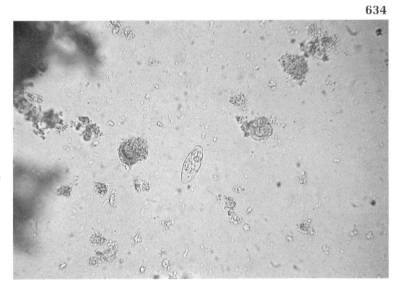

635

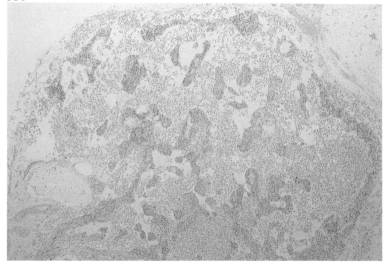

636

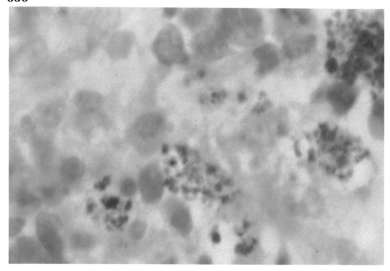

635 and **636**   **Acquired immune deficiency syndrome.** Section of a mesenteric lymph node of a patient with AIDS. **635** shows that many of the lymphocytes have disappeared, leaving a 'washed out' appearance. The expanded sinusoids contain pale-staining macrophages. **636** is a high-power photograph obtained after staining the sinusoidal macrophages by the Ziehl–Neelsen method. Numerous acid-fast bacilli are seen. Their morphology differs from that of *Mycobacterium tuberculosis* in that they are shorter and more slender. Infections resulting from these atypical mycobacteria are resistant to standard anti-tuberculous therapy.

INDEX

INDEX

References are to page numbers

Virchow's node   53

Worm infestation   201-207